Negotiating Mistrust

CONTEMPORARY ETHNOGRAPHY

Alma Gottlieb and Timothy R. Landry, *Series Editors*

A complete list of books in the series
is available from the publisher.

# NEGOTIATING MISTRUST

Patients and Healers Across Traditional, Islamic,
and Biomedical Health Sectors of Niger

Scott M. Youngstedt

**PENN**

UNIVERSITY OF PENNSYLVANIA PRESS

PHILADELPHIA

Published by
University of Pennsylvania Press
Philadelphia, Pennsylvania 19104–4112 USA
www.pennpress.org

EU Authorized Representative: Easy Access System
Europe—Mustamäe tee 50, 10621 Tallinn, Estonia,
gpsr.requests@easproject.com.

Printed in the United States of America on acid-free paper
10 9 8 7 6 5 4 3 2 1

A Cataloging-in-Publication record is
available from the Library of Congress

Paperback ISBN 978-1-5128-2882-5
Hardback ISBN 978-1-5128-2883-2
eBook ISBN 978-1-5128-2884-9

*To Brian Nowak*

# CONTENTS

# ILLUSTRATIONS

## Maps

## Tables

## Figures

# INTRODUCTION

## Mariama's Quest for Health

Mariama, a Hausa woman, grew up in a typical small village without a primary school near Maradi in south central Niger. Now 57 years old, she has lived in Niamey, the capital city of the Republic of Niger, since she was 20. Mariama's beautiful round ebony face is marked on either side with two three-centimeter vertical traditional scarification patterns that she received as a child, while deep smile lines together with furrows on her forehead and bloodshot eyes reflect a life of joy and of hardship—of marriage and rearing three children, of divorce and remarriage, of three miscarriages, of fostering her sister's children for years and helping to raise her grandchildren, of hours cooking over wood fires in poorly ventilated traditional kitchens, and of pain. Her frequent captivating smiles and laughter are highlighted by bright white, perfectly straight teeth, even though she has never sought dental care and has relied more on traditional neem chewing sticks than toothbrushes and toothpaste, and because, unlike many Nigériens, she never developed a taste for heavily sugared tea or kola nuts.

Mariama's face also reveals long-term physical pain that has plagued her for years. Mariama operated a small restaurant offering spectacularly complex and delicious meals for many years until about 10 years ago, when her occasional full body aches worsened and became chronic, compelling her to retire. Her mother, sisters, and friends diagnosed her ailment as arthritis, partly because Mariama suffers the most during the cool season. This "therapy management group" (Janzen 1978) regularly gives Mariama a wide assortment of traditional plant medicines as well as biomedical drugs. Indeed, Nigériens commonly share a variety of types of medication with family and friends.

"Therapy management groups" consisting of family, friends, and neighbors "are at the heart of African healing" (Feierman and Janzen 1992, 18). In Niger,

as elsewhere in Africa, these groups help make diagnoses of the patient's illness and suggest or offer treatments. They help choose healers and sometimes visit healers together with the patient. Mariama's therapy management
group was not hierarchically organized, but some groups are—for example,
those that organize therapy for children. Therapy management groups also
provide supportive care such as emotional support, helping with chores, or
bringing food to a hospitalized patient because public hospitals in Niger do
not offer meals. Mariama and her medical team, like most people in Niamey,
purchase medicine primarily from mobile ambulatory street vendors of traditional plant medicine and other itinerant street healers who sell a full range
of pharmaceutical drugs. Dozens of these street vendors can be found every
day on the busy street just a block from Mariama's home and one lives right
next door. Mariama and her team occasionally visit formal sector pharmacies
as well.

Mariama's husband, Abdourahmane, worries about this mixing of multiple medicines. Abdourahmane, now 64 years old, is an educated man who
identifies as Hausa, even though his father is Kanuri and his mother is
Fulani.[1] He was once an airplane mechanic but has been mostly unemployed
for 35 years after suffering chemical poisoning while working on a crop
duster for the Ministry of Agriculture. (I will revisit Abdourahmane and the
ways that he has handled his own health crises later in the book.) When I
asked him about Mariama's many treatments, he explained, "Mariama and
her family and friends have good intentions, but they have no idea what
they are doing. None of them have been to school, so they cannot read labels
on medicines that include dosage information and warnings. She just takes
whatever they give her, and sometimes she seems to get temporary relief and
other times she seems worse off. But Mariama is really suffering, so I cannot
really fault her for trying to do something about it." His words encompass a
common refrain in discussions about medicine in Niger; while many question their efficacy and people's ability to take them properly, many men and
women are resigned to the fact that none of the options available to them
may be viable.

At one point in her long quest for healing, Mariama became convinced
that she was victim of witchcraft perpetrated by a restaurant competitor
or an angry customer to whom she denied credit. Abdourahmane told her
that this is *maganar banza* (foolish talk), that witches are just an African
superstition, and that good Muslims do not believe in such things. Mariama

countered Abdourahmane's argument by informing him that she had in fact purchased anti-witch medicine in an Islamic medicine shop and by explaining that "Except for the white skin, the witch on the label looks a lot like the way my parents described them to me." She considers herself a good Muslim who always completes her daily prayers, fasts during Ramadan, and recently exchanged her traditional, colorful, floral headscarves for plain black hijab, following a trend that emerged about a dozen years ago in Niamey alongside reformist Islamist movements. Mariama saw no contradiction in trying some anti-witch incense for a week despite her husband's admonitions. She said it failed to provide her any relief.

After years of suffering, Abdourahmane and Mariama saved enough money for a visit to a private biomedical clinic seeking a diagnosis and therapy options for Mariama. The consultation cost them 15,000 CFA (about 30 USD), or about 10 days' worth of living expenses for the two of them together.[2] After a battery of tests, the physician informed Mariama that she has sickle cell trait and that there is no way to cure it. Sickle cell trait is a genetic blood disorder. Most who have it are asymptomatic, but some experience pain crises. Recognizing the couple's poverty, the physician recommended that she rest and take paracetamol or ibuprofen during particularly painful episodes. Mariama received this news with a mixture of stoicism and skepticism. As she reflected, "It is good to know what I have, but I still think that I might find ways to treat it or even cure it."

Indeed, Mariama has continued to pursue many options. In addition to continuing to accept many traditional and pharmaceutical medications from her family and friends, two years ago, upon the recommendation of her brother, she traveled to Diffa—a city in southeastern Niger, 1,500 kilometers from Niamey—to visit a renowned traditional healer of Kanuri ethnicity who works with spirits and plants. Mariama received gifts and loans and she and Abdourahmane spent all their money to cover the cost of this venture, which amounted to about 90,000 CFA with 80,000 CFA for bus tickets, a 5,000 CFA healer's fee, and other expenses—or six times what she spent to see the biomedical specialist. Mariama feels most uncomfortable sitting, yet she was willing to sit on a crowded bus for two days each way of her long journey, a willingness that further signals her commitment to finding relief. She was also willing to travel to a very dangerous city; Diffa has been under siege from the infamous Boko Haram terrorist group, and authorities have imposed a dusk-to-dawn curfew for the past few years. The healer diagnosed

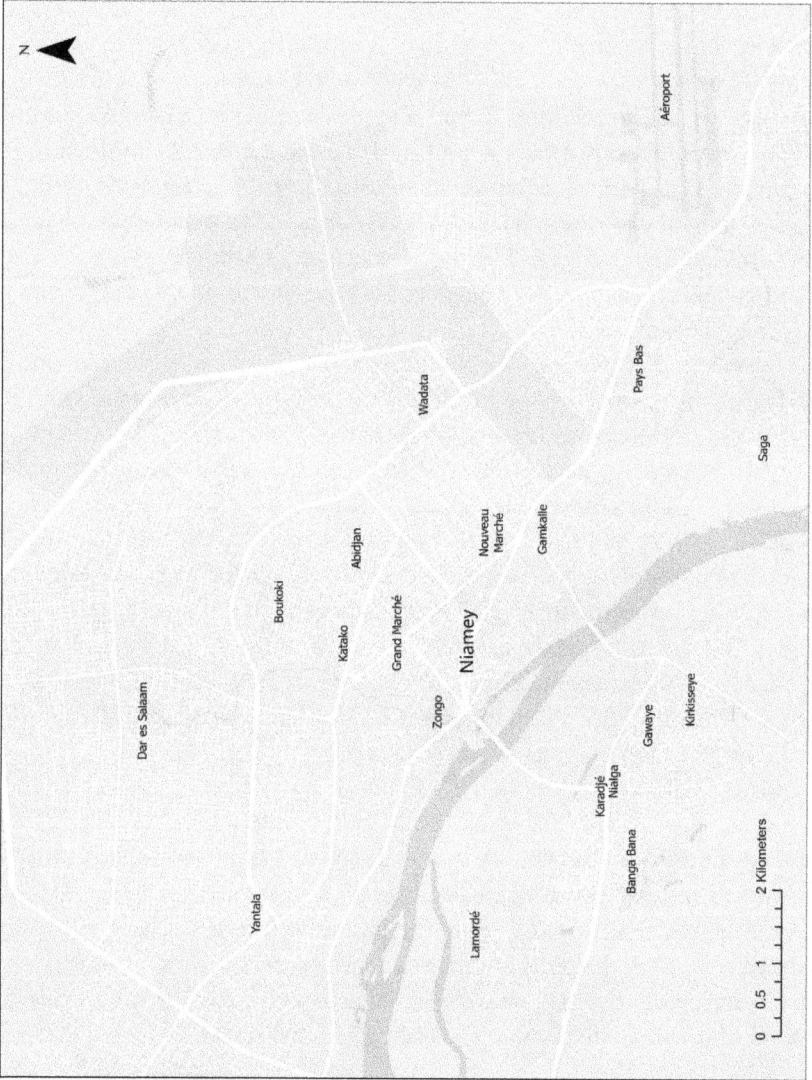

Map I.1. Niamey neighborhoods. Map by Madeline S. Payne.

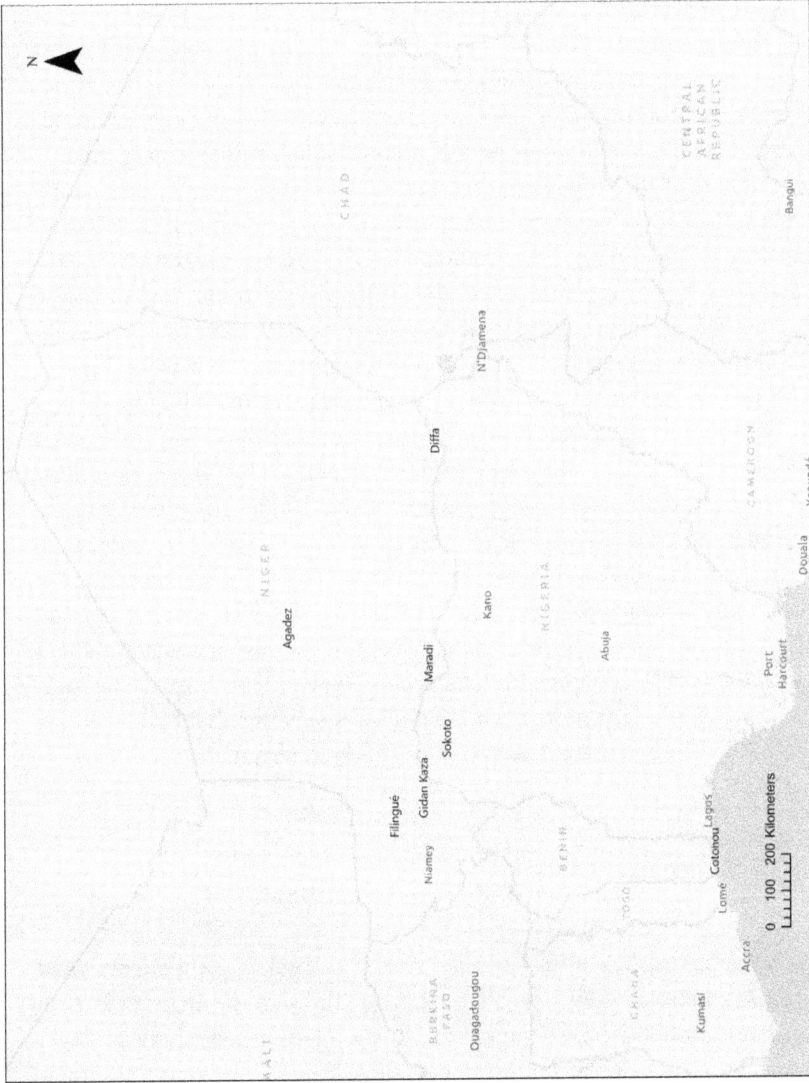

Map I.2. West Africa. Map by Madeline S. Payne.

Mariama's suffering as due to the attack of an angry spirit, and he treated it with herbal medicine. When Mariama returned to Niamey, she reported that she felt great for about three weeks. And she looked good, with a spring in her step that I had not seen for a long time. Then, her debilitating pain returned.

Mariama's therapeutic trajectory is unique while simultaneously broadly representative of the strategies and sentiments of Nigériens who commonly use all three of Niger's primary health care sectors—traditional, Islamic, and biomedical—sequentially and simultaneously. Mariama sought a biomedical diagnosis of her condition but relies primarily on traditional medicine from multiple ethnic groups to treat it, as do many Nigériens. Mariama's reliance on therapy management groups is also typical, as is her willingness to accept and try medicines that have been gifted to her, including medicines that she would never have purchased or tried on her own. The widespread mistrust of folk healers and their medicines expressed by Nigériens is illustrated in Abdourahmane's concerns, and in the debates between Mariama and Abdourahmane about witches and Islamic medicine. My synopsis of Mariama's situation also reveals the importance of the material culture of packaging in decision-making, since she and many others feel that images on medication containers can help them discern important information about the purposes of the contents. Mariama's perpetual and costly quest for healing, even in the face of news from biomedical specialists that her condition is uncurable, also illustrates a common relentless determination to seek well-being in Niger.

## The Aim and Focus of the Book

*Negotiating Mistrust* examines a wide diversity of healers and patients—and interactions between them—in Niamey, Niger, through the analytical prism of mistrust. I offer a holistic approach to the medical landscape in Niger by focusing on the intersections among three medical sectors: traditional, Islamic, and biomedical. My broad-stroke analysis simultaneously emphasizes the lived experiences of health, illness, and therapy of real people. "Traditional medicine" is the term used in local languages by Nigériens—and by me—to describe local Nigérien concepts of health, illness, and healing as well as therapies involving plants, minor surgeries, and spirits. My use of the term "Islamic medicine" is expansive, as it includes knowledge of health and therapeutics found in the Qur'an and the Hadiths (sayings of the Prophet

Muhammad) as well as concepts without Islamic theological foundations that have been absorbed by Muslim communities over time, such as Greek humoral ideas. Nigériens debate what is and what is not "Islamic medicine." "Biomedicine," or "allopathic medicine," involves the scientific application of the principles of biology and biochemistry to medical research and practice. Biomedical healthcare professionals prevent and treat diseases with industrially manufactured medications and vaccines as well as minor and major surgeries. Nigériens typically refer to biomedicine as "modern medicine" or "hospital medicine." I will define these medical sectors with much more precision and nuance in Chapter 1.

I focus on Nigériens' pervasive mistrust of medicines and therapies, healers, and local and global health care institutions across traditional, Islamic, and biomedical sectors, as well as the strategies that healers and health care institutions employ in efforts to generate medical trust, for three reasons. First, I argue that nuanced analysis of the interplay between mistrust and trust is key to understanding the decisions that health-seeking Nigériens make among the multiple options available to them, while recognizing that in one of the world's very poorest countries, many forms of biomedical health care—and some traditional and Islamic medicine—are unaffordable to most people. Furthermore, I will show the interrelationship between medical pluralism and medical mistrust.

Second, medical mistrust is relatively understudied and usually not the focus of studies, despite its central importance in health care contexts. Rather than simplistically viewing medical mistrust in Niger as pathological, I will argue and marshal evidence to demonstrate that mistrust and trust are not mutually exclusive and usually not absolute but exist on a fluid continuum, involve cognitive and affective dimensions, and are shaped by particular historical, contemporary, and personal contexts. Furthermore, drawing from Nigérien perspectives and cultural theory, I will argue that medical mistrust often functions as a pragmatic, defensive attitude of engagement with uncertainty (Luhmann 2014), "intersecting precarities" (MacGregor et al. 2021), and risk (Douglas 1992). Mistrust complicates medical decision-making, but Nigériens are not paralyzed by it. While I emphasize the productivity of medical mistrust, I also recognize that it can be source of great frustration for Nigériens and others who want to trust their health care providers, and that medical mistrust can have lethal consequences for public health.

Third, medical mistrust in various forms is widespread, and probably universal. My focused study of the medical mistrust–trust dynamic in Niger can yield important insights on health care dynamics in the United States or anywhere. Medical mistrust emerges particularly in times of uncertainty, and we are living in "liquid times" (Bauman 2007) of "post-truth" (Mühlfried 2018, 16), disinformation, fakery, artificial intelligence, and waning confidence in science and governments.

Nigériens are not generally mistrustful, but medical mistrust is deep-rooted and widespread in Niger for reasons this book will elucidate. No occupation, except for politician or state official, is stigmatized as charlatanism in the way the healing occupation is in Niamey. Despite pervasive mistrust of medical systems and institutions, medicines, and healers of all sectors for diverse historical reasons, tens of thousands of Nigériens consult with and purchase medicines from healers daily on the streets of Niamey because their determination to get well helps them overcome their skepticism. Since people in Niamey are often mistrustful of medical care—sometimes even of all three sectors—practitioners must exert enormous energy earning potential patients' trust. They do this in a variety of ways, but for the street practitioners who are the focus of this book, the manipulation of the material culture of medicine (through marketing and packaging) is one of the key means through which they seek to garner and retain clients. Each medical sector had a historical point of arrival in Niamey, and each remains and flourishes. Chapter 1 traces the history of medical pluralism in Niamey and briefly introduces the reasons for widespread mistrust of each sector as well as the links between pluralism and mistrust. Chapter 3 analyzes the historical origins and contemporary reality of medical mistrust in more detail.

Seeking health care in Niger involves navigating medical pluralism, uncertainty and mistrust, financial obstacles, and poor access to quality biomedical services. The stakes of finding medical relief are high in a context where health and life itself are precarious. Colonialism, state mismanagement, global neoliberalism, structural adjustment, and neocolonialism have inflicted structural violence on Nigériens, relegating Niger to a status at—or very near—the bottom of the United Nations Human Development Index for decades (UNDP 2022). More than one-half of Nigériens live in "extreme poverty" (World Bank 2024). This toxic combination of factors prevents Nigériens for accessing human rights, including the right to adequate health care. This book will contribute to a deeper understanding of how people make medical decisions in precarious environments where multiple therapeutic options are available but where, to many people, many options are unaffordable and few seem

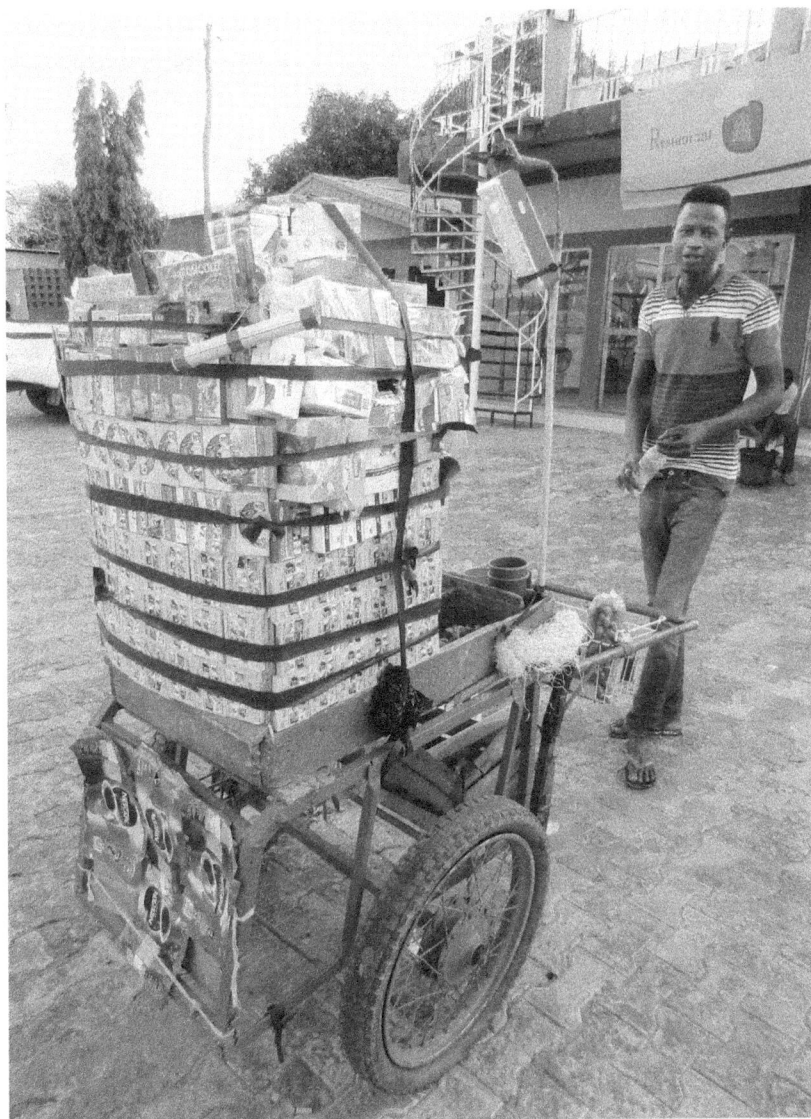

Figure I.1. Itinerant pharmaceutical vendor with medical tower on pushcart. Photo by author.

promising. The book will also advance understanding about what creates contextualized medical mistrust and how it shapes patients' decision-making as well as healers' strategies in the face of mistrust.

Traditional, Islamic, and biomedical health sectors in Niger are rapidly changing, and are increasingly intertwined and influencing each other. I make the case that to develop a holistic understanding of Niger's healing cultures, we need to explore overlapping medical sectors and the factors that influence patients' decisions within and across them. By analyzing them together, *Negotiating Mistrust* provides insight into the interplay of key Africanist medical and cultural anthropological analytical concerns, including how people navigate medical pluralism, the dialectical tension between mistrust and trust, and ways that the material culture of medicine is a powerful means through which healers assert and reinforce their legitimacy as well as an important variable in patients' decision-making. Because multiple forms of healing are increasingly accessible globally, this book provides important insights into how they influence each other and how people navigate therapeutic options on the fly—especially through the informal sector—based on pragmatic issues such as availability and affordability, as well as symbolic dimensions such as social identities and affiliations and social distances between patients and healers. In addition, I make the counterintuitive argument that the widespread mistrust of healers is partly why three somewhat separate—yet increasingly overlapping—medical sectors are changing, adapting, and flourishing in Niger.

While this book focuses on Niger, it addresses crucial issues that are not confined to Niger or Africa in general. We can learn something from the Nigérien context that helps us better understand medical mistrust and medical pluralism in our own lives. After all, one of the key goals of anthropology is "making the strange familiar and the familiar strange." In the U.S.—where biomedicine reigns supreme as much as anywhere in the world—millions of people mistrust physicians, vaccinations, pills, and science in general, and their numbers are growing. A widely circulating rumor in the U.S. over the last few years is that scientists can cure cancer, but there is much more money to be made treating it (Worldwide Cancer Research 2020). Furthermore, millions of Americans try various alternatives to biomedicine, including herbal supplements that are not approved by the FDA, crystals, acupuncture, prayers, remedies advertised on television, and cannabis. Medical pluralism and medical mistrust are found around the world—including the poorest and wealthiest countries—for overlapping reasons, as well as very different reasons of sociohistorical context.

In this work, I focus on the careers of generalist healers of all three sectors who work on the street and in everyday markets and in small, stand-alone boutiques. Thousands operate on Niamey's streets. Most are ambulatory and carry sacks or "medicine towers" perched atop their heads or use wheelbarrows or pushcarts. By "generalist healers" I mean healers who typically treat 30 or more problems, everything from headaches and colds to malaria and cancer. There is a great amount of overlap in the ailments treated by traditional, Islamic, and biomedical healers, but only traditional and Islamic healers deal with problems caused by spirits, witches, and sorcerers. I use the term "healer" very broadly, to include everyone from old traditional healers who come from families of healers who consider healing their life calling to young, mobile vendors of pharmaceutical drugs who primarily consider themselves as entrepreneurs.

Almost all generalist healers on the streets of Niamey are men. There are many women healers in Niamey as well—especially herbalists who work to ensure women's fertility—but almost all work from the privacy of their homes or their clients' homes. One important exception to this is women street healers who sell medicine to treat "heat." They are probably the single most common type of healers on the streets of Niamey. These women thus form an important part of my analysis, especially in my extended discussion in Chapter 2 of "heat"–"cold"—a local and regional illness complex. Clients of generalist healers are roughly evenly split between men and women.

I chose this emphasis first, because these are the most commonly used therapies in Niamey, and second, to differentiate this study from most other scholarship on health, illness, and healing in Niger and Northern Nigeria. Several scholars address the entanglements of pluralistic medical sectors in the lives of healers and/or patients, including especially Conerly Casey (2021), Barbara M. Cooper (2019), Murray Last (1992), Adeline Masquelier (2001), Susan Rasmussen (2001), and Kelley Sams (2017). I draw from these crucial works—and others[3]—and build on them by contributing understanding of how the trust–mistrust dyad offers a generative entry point into the study of medical pluralism and the fluidity between sectors. Much of this extant scholarship focuses on healing consultations and treatments provided: (1) in the "private" spaces of public and private hospitals and clinics and within people's compounds;[4] (2) in single ethnic groups, such as Fulani,[5] Hausa,[6] Mawri,[7] Songhay-Zarma,[8] Tuareg,[9] and Azawagh Arabs;[10] (3) in rural settings;[11] or

Table I.1. Types of Medicines in Niamey's Informal Sector

| Category | Traditional | Islamic | Biomedical |
|---|---|---|---|
| Supernatural | 32 evil spirits, djinn, sorcery & witchcraft | 9 sihir<br>8 bewitchment<br>7 bad spirits<br>3 sayful jini<br>2 ilajis sihir (evil spirit) | |
| Panaceas    water | | 11 Zam Zam (water)<br>7 healing water<br>4 mineral water<br>3 miracle water | |
|            incense | | 14 Qur'anic incense<br>1 incense | |
|            honey | | 9 Qur'anic honey<br>6 honey | |
|            plant | | 5 habatou saouda | |
| Digestive and Gastrointestinal | 18 intestinal<br>17 gastric ulcers<br>12 hemorrhoids<br>9 abdominal<br>6 kidney<br>5 bladder | 6 Costus | 9 Cimetidine (ulcers) |
| Pain Management | 19 dental<br>15 aches and pains<br>5 headaches, migraines | 4 Parimol | 37 Paracetamol<br>32 Ibuprofen/Ibucap<br>28 Efferalgen<br>17 Really Extra<br>11 Socomol<br>6 Diclofenac<br>9 Niffuril (arthritis) |
| Metabolic, Endocrine and Liver | 14 hypertension<br>13 diabetes<br>8 jaundice | | 12 Coartem (malaria) |
| Reproductive | 8 love, sex, pregnancy and postpartum | 5 libido and sperm<br>2 Super Bazouka<br>1 penile enlargement<br>2 pregnancy | 5 Venegra (erectile dysfunction) |

| Category | Traditional | Islamic | Biomedical |
|---|---|---|---|
| Dermatological and Topical | 10 itching<br>7 hemacie | 11 Qur'anic pomades<br>4 pomades<br>8 olive oil (El Madinah)<br>3 Argan oil<br>2 Nugreek oil<br>2 Mai ayu<br>8 plant-based soap and shampoo<br>5 Zabat cream | |
| Infectious Disease | 8 STDs (6), AIDS (2)<br>6 typhoid | | 20 Amoxycilline<br>14 Flagyl<br>11 Doxacilline<br>8 Metronidazole |
| Cold Relief | | | 17 Kold Time<br>16 Mixagrip<br>10 Medic<br>6 Komix |
| Sensory and Cognitive | 5 hearing | 3 memory improvement,<br>3 mal kwando<br>3 allugaton<br>3 amber | |
| Pediatric | 10 children, including "walking medicine" | | |

Table by Warren K. Fincher.

(4) for specific health challenges such as pregnancy and childbirth,[12] fistula,[13] polio,[14] and spirit possession.[15]

This book, in contrast, focuses on multiethnic and transethnic medical interactions between healers and patients across three overlapping therapeutic traditions involving a vast range of health conditions—from everyday ailments to life-threating problems—that occur on streets of Niamey, which is by far Niger's biggest city. I also consider health, illness, and healing discussions and therapies as they take place in the privacy of people's homes.

The patients and healers who are the focus of this book are representative of the ethnolinguistic diversity of Niamey, which consists of about 40 percent Hausa, 40 percent Zarma-Songhay,[16] 5 percent Fulani, 5 percent Tuareg, 4 percent Mawri, and small numbers of other ethnolinguistic groups of Niger and other countries in the region.[17]

While my focus is on the three major therapeutic sectors—traditional, Islamic, and biomedical—several micro healing communities also exist in Niamey, including Chinese, Christian, Baha'i, and Hindu. Chinese traditional medicine is the only one that has generated interest outside of its own community in Niamey, partly because it is the only one that has "tried" to lure patients—or more precisely, it is the only one whose healers and entrepreneurs, both Chinese and Nigérien, have tried to gain clients—and partly because of its reputation for emphasizing powerful, natural herbs in healing. Despite awareness of the fringes of the therapeutic landscape in Niamey, I will not be focusing on these practices due to their lack of prevalence among Nigériens.

## The Ethos of Health and Well-Being in Niger: *Lahiya Ta Hi Kud'i*

One day in 2021 while listening with a streetside conversation group in Niamey to the Hausa language program of Radio France Internationale (RFI), I heard the announcer use the adage *lahiya ta hi kud'i*, or health is more important than money. I recognized it as clever spin on *Gaskiya Ta Fi Kwabo*, the name of first Hausa language newspaper, which has been published three times a week since 1937 in Kano, Nigeria, and which means figuratively, "the truth is more important than money." Masquelier (2001, 77) similarly showed that for the Mawri of Niger, "Health is the most important thing that one can have." Recall that Mariama and Abdourahmane spent all their money and incurred debt to seek traditional therapy for an ailment that biomedical specialists deemed incurable. My conversation partners readily agreed with the expression, variations of which are used in many languages around the world. However, 60-year-old Dogo complicated the discussion by adding, "But sometimes it is hard to be healthy if one cannot afford good food, clean water, and medicine." He recognized that poverty and structural violence are barriers to health.

Health and well-being are always on the minds and tongues of Nigériens. Greetings are an incredibly important element of everyday life and etiquette in Niger. Most Nigériens greet dozens of people daily, and their greetings usually involve several back-and-forth questions and responses, unlike the simple "How are you?" that is common in the U.S. Proper and polite greetings are a simple but important affirmation of humanity and exchanging them is one consistent pleasure of life in Niger. I use many Hausa terms in the text because it is the most is the most widely spoken language in Niamey (along with Zarma), and it is the local language that I speak. Across the languages of Niger and throughout the Sahel, the most common greetings involve asking about the current state of health and well-being of individuals, families, compounds, and even whole cities. In addition, Nigériens also use greetings that are specific to the health of the body. For example, the Hausa ask "*Ina jiki?*" (How is your body?), the Zarma ask "*Mate gaham?*" (How is your body? or literally, How is the meat on you?), and the Fulani ask "*Jam bandu?*" (Is your body at peace or healthy?). Nigériens almost always offer the formulaic response that "all is well"—regardless of their actual condition. More specifically, all Nigérien languages include a complex, polysemic word or short phrase that refers, depending on context, to "health," "well-being," "peace," or "prosperity" (or all of these holistically), that is used in response to greetings. In Hausa, the word is *lahiya* (usually accompanied by *lau* [very]), in Zarma, *baani*; in Fulfulde, *jam*; in Tamashek, *alheri* (always accompanied by *ras* [only]); in Gourmance, *lafia*; in Kanuri, *klewa*; and in Toubou, *wasa*. Once these greetings are completed, people may then discuss the actual state of their health with close family and friends.

A paradox animates the ethos of health and healing, and life and death in Niamey: The coexistence of a pervasive patient, stoic attitude toward and seemingly fatalistic acceptance of illness, disease, and death, alongside the life-long creative pursuit of health and well-being. Some years ago, anthropologist Paul Stoller (2004, 90) argued that in Niger illness is regarded as a normal condition, "an ever-present companion" that people seek to address through "acceptance, pragmatism, and patience." These attitudes are expressed in concrete behaviors. Historian Barbara Cooper (2019, 164) documented that people of Sahelian cultures in general and Nigérien cultures in particular highly value the endurance of pain. Nigérien women historically and in the present typically endure labor and childbirth alone and silently. Nigérien men typically are highly reluctant to complain about their illnesses. In most Nigérien cultures, death and funerals are recognized quietly and stoically and emphasize acceptance of Allah's will. People pray that Allah will forgive their deceased family and friends for any of their shortcomings and offer simple greetings to that effect. Indeed, the pervasiveness of Islam today in Niger—98 percent of the population in Muslim—certainly contributes to this acceptance of illness and death; however, as Mariama's example reminds us, this does not mean that people do not try relentlessly to improve their health. Alongside a fatalistic attitude regarding illness and misfortune, Nigérien Muslims also acknowledge human agency. They believe that for each ailment, Allah created a remedy, and that people can learn these remedies through careful study of the Qur'an.

Nigériens typically define health as more just the absence of illness or disease, and they understand it much more globally than biomedicine typically does (Baronov 2008; Jaffré and Olivier de Sardan 2003; Roberts 2021; Stoller 2004; Wall, 1988). For example, the Nigérien Hausa word *lahiya* refers to "proper ordering, correct structuring, and general well-being of the social order and the individual's relations within it, as well as the state of the wellness in the human body" (Wall 1988, 211). It can also refer to balance in one's relationships with Allah and/or the spirit world. It thus does not narrowly refer to the body, but rather it links physical well-being with the well-being of the wider society and an individual's place within it. As this term suggests, Nigériens view social, spiritual, and physical health as interconnected—being out of balance in one dimension of life can lead to imbalances in others. In contrast with wellness of the body, are pain (*ciwo*) and injury or disrupted function (*cuta*). The Hausa word *magani* means "medicine," "remedy," and more broadly "that which restores order." The various usages of the term reflect how wellness is seen as both important and broad: coolness is the *magani* for too much heat in the body; a patch is the *magani* for a flat tire; resolving a dispute peacefully is the *magani* for social disharmony. Other Nigérien languages have similar polysemic terms.

In sum, well-being matters a lot to Nigériens. However, maintaining physical health and recovering from or at least managing illnesses in Niger is elusive given rapid and often disruptive social change, grinding poverty, intersecting precarities, and complex overlapping medical sectors.

## Self-Care and Therapy Management Groups in Nigérien Pluralist Medicine

In addition to consulting with thousands of healers across three medical sectors, many Nigériens consider themselves healers supported by a team of healers. That is, an enormous amount of medical care in Niamey is self-care involving home remedies and grandparents' recipes and the advice and medicine shared by "therapy management groups" (Janzen 1978) consisting of family and close friends. Many Nigériens see informal street traditional, Islamic, and biomedical vendors as the sources of the raw materials to create their own home concoctions. Indeed, many—perhaps most—encounters between clients and healers on the streets of Niamey are simple business transactions because clients have already diagnosed themselves and decided on courses of treatment before these encounters take place. Nigériens in Niamey typically are very knowledgeable about local plants and trees and their purported medicinal properties—especially if they were born in or have spent significant time in rural areas of Niger. In 2023, together with research assistants I collected and photographed 35 plant medicines. When I shared these photographs with my Nigérien interlocutors, on average they could identify more than 95 percent of them. They are also widely familiar with "traditional" Islamic medicines and therapies as well as the most common pharmaceutical drugs sold by mobile vendors.

Home-based medical self-care is common across Africa. For example, in *Sharing the Burden of Sickness: A History of Healing and Medicine in Accra*, Jonathan Roberts (2021, 6–7) identifies "the common-sense practice of self-healing with herbal remedies and over-the-counter medicines" as the fifth therapeutic tradition in Accra, separate from West African, Islamic, Christian, and Western traditions. While I recognize the importance of self-care in Niamey, I do not consider it a separate sector. However, it is key to unpacking core themes of this book. The reality that nearly everyone considers themselves as healers of sorts contributes to medical pluralism and medical mistrust. Although Nigériens use therapies across all three medical sectors simultaneously and sequentially, many Nigériens prefer one sector over the others. Among Nigériens, trust and social distance are intertwined. The greater the social distance, the more likely that people are mistrusted. One trusts oneself above all others, followed by an inner circle of family and friends. Unlike most Westerners, Nigériens have not ceded authority to credentialed medical providers.

## Methodological Strategies, Perspectives, and a Note on Words

I was drawn to conduct a focused study of health and well-being and healing beginning in 2017 after a long ethnographic career in Niger that began in 1988 and has included 25 visits. Although my early work did not explicitly focus on health and healing, these topics were frequently in the background of my research and were important parts of my interlocuters' lives. My early and longtime research focused on social well-being, documented in my book *Surviving with Dignity: Hausa Communities of Niamey, Niger* (2013). I realize now more than ever that Nigériens regard socio-emotional well-being as integral to overall health. During my first visit in 1988, I realized that health and healing were a very important part of life in Niger. That year, I was invited to a spirit possession ceremony—where I initially learned about the importance of spirits in healing—and I have been to many others since then. My survey of the occupations of Hausa migrants in Niamey in the early 1990s included interviews with several traditional and Islamic healers. I have also remained in continuous contact since 1991 with several men and their extended families. As our friendships deepened over the years, some became comfortable sharing intimate details of their health trajectories with me long before I initiated this project.

From 2011 to 2018 my collaborative ethnographic research with cultural geographer Sara Beth Keough focused on multiple dimensions of water in Niamey, culminating with the publication of *Water, Life, and Profit: Fluid Economies and Cultures of Niamey, Niger* (2019). The book included analysis of the problems that poor Nigériens face in accessing clean water and the serious health implications involved, adding depth to the expression "water is life," an adage used in Nigérien languages and nearly universally around the world. When I informed accomplished medical anthropologist and longtime friend Rachel Chapman of my current work, she declared, "You have been a medical anthropologist all along, you just did not know it!" She was onto something, though I might be more accurately described as a cultural anthropologist who studies medicine.

In this book, I rely primarily on six rounds of ethnographic research in 2017, 2018, 2019, 2021, 2022, and 2023 spanning a total of 10 months, though I also draw from my earlier studies as well as the literature on health, illness, and healing in Niger, West Africa, and beyond, as I have done in this introduction. My research focused on talking with healers and patients and listening to their stories as well as focused observations and participant observation. I spent much of my time hanging out in informal streetside *hira* (conversation groups)—as I always have done when I am in Niamey—participating in the natural flow of dialogue while also finding occasions to steer the talk toward health and healing. From the vantage point of my favorite *hira* group, I was able to observe interactions between healers of all sectors and their clients any time I spent more than 30 minutes there, which was almost every day, and sometimes all three were simultaneously in view. In addition, I engaged in participant observation in many people's homes, where I was exposed to some of the ways that families make decisions about therapies and administer medicines. I also draw from my own engagement with traditional, Islamic, and biomedicine in Niamey as over the years I have faced colds, nosebleeds during the harmattan season when dry winds kick up sand from the Sahara, a severely sprained ankle, amoebic dysentery, malaria, and a mysterious ailment that defied biomedical diagnosis and that was worse than all the others. I learned from these experiences about how a variety of medicines feel when taken, and more broadly about the precarity of health in Niger and people's willingness, including my own, to try new and different things despite skepticism, in an effort to feel better.

I also engaged in formally structured fieldwork, more specifically: (1) I interviewed healers and patients in all three primary medical sectors—a total of 126 healers (42 traditional herbalists, 24 Islamic pharmacists and marabouts, 67 informal vendors of pharmaceuticals) and 120 patients; (2) I gathered six "health life histories"; and (3) I met multiple times over several years with three focus groups consisting of six to eight—somewhat stable but also rotating—people each. In addition, (4) I attended l'Association des Tradi-Practiciens du Niger (Association of Traditional Medical Practitioners or ATPN) meetings and interviewed its Board of Directors, (5) I analyzed the material culture of medicines themselves as well as the marketing of medicines through written labeling and imagery across medical sectors in physical form on the streets of Niamey as well as in social media, websites, and radio and television programs, and (6) I used photography to document the working environments of healers and the material culture of medical packaging and medicine.

(1) Interviews with healers focused on careers in the profession, means of acquiring knowledge, the range of ailments treated, and interactions with other healers within and across medical systems. Interviews with patients focused on range of factors in decision-making, the range of ailments for which treatment is sought, and satisfaction with services and medicines received. The interviews were structured, but I allowed participants opportunities to speak extemporaneously so that they could discuss healing topics that were meaningful to them. They typically lasted about 20 to 30 minutes each, though some were much longer. I recorded these verbatim by hand,

mostly in Hausa, though some in French. Most Zarma-Songhay in Niamey speak Hausa or French. At times when the pace of answers was too much for me, I simply translated them directly into English. Two research assistants also administered interviews, particularly in Fulfulde and Tamashek—languages of the Fulani and Tuareg that I do not speak—and transcribed them in Hausa or French for my benefit. I also recorded the ethnicity, gender, age, class, education, and neighborhoods of healers, and incorporated these data in analyses.

(2) The health life histories allowed people to freely discuss health trajectories over their life spans. I used very few prompts, and I only occasionally interrupted to ask for details that seemed missing. The participants are people that I have known for at least a few years, others I have known for decades, and two for 32 years. I audio-recorded three of these with permission and recorded the others by hand. These lasted from one hour to a few hours and in some cases many more. (3) My focus group discussions were mostly open-ended, free-flowing, and spontaneous, after typically opening with a prompt from me, such as "What kinds of medicines do you have at home today?" or "What do you think about the new Islamic medicine shop in your neighborhood?" (4) I spoke with the Board of Directors of the Association des Tradi-Practiciens du Niger (ATPN) to gain understanding the association's history, membership, objectives, and challenges. I also observed traditional practitioners sharing ideas about diverse medicines and how to interact with patients to build trust. (5) I observed and documented dozens of medicines—and packaging labels and inserts—across all three medical sectors, noting local names, appearances, aromas, shapes, and therapeutic uses. I was particularly interested in observing the ways that healers display medicines. (6) I used photography to document healers and their collections of medicines, especially on the street but also in small shops.

My primary aim is to shed light on the meanings Nigériens give to their health, illness, and healing experiences. However, I also consider biomedical understandings of "disease," or "health-related afflictions linked to biological pathologies" (Baronov 2008, 126). Making sense of the Nigérien lived experiences is difficult even when it involves different views of the natural world, as I will explain in Chapter 2 in the case of the "heat"–"cold" complex. Even more challenging is representing and interpreting the supernatural worlds of Nigériens involving spirits, sorcery, witchcraft, and magic, for misunderstandings of supernatural knowledge and practices lie at the very heart of the most pernicious and unproductive stereotypes of Africa as the irrational and/or evil Dark Continent. Nigériens are as rational and as irrational in their thoughts regarding health and other important life matters as any people in the world, and their understandings and experiences of health, illness, and healing can only be understood in cultural and sociohistorical context and by keeping an open mind. In addition to aiming to understand cultural differences, in *Negotiating Mistrust* I will show some of the important ways that Nigériens are navigating decisions and concerns that are widespread around the world if not universals; it is "possible to find common ground across cultural difference" (Falen 2018, 5). These include making choices among and between medical sectors, balancing self-care and the advice of family and friends with ceding therapeutic authority to some professional healers but not others, and facing medical skepticism, doubt, fear, and mistrust. Anthropology can help us understand others and with reflection facilitates deeper understanding of ourselves and offers valuable perspectives for comprehending these contemporary troubled times of war, climate disruption, and pandemics in which confidence in science and biomedicine, governments, and international institutions is in decline globally.

I conclude with a few notes on word usages. I use many Hausa terms because of the widespread use of Hausa in Niger, and because more scholars have written about Hausa health and medicine than that of other ethnic groups in Niger and neighboring Northern Nigeria. I also use terms from other Nigérien languages when appropriate, for example when interviewees or other scholars do so. Following France's colonial policy, with very few exceptions schools in independent Niger have never taught literacy in Nigérien languages. Thus, there are no standardized ways of writing Hausa in Niger. The very few Nigériens who write informally or formally in Hausa seem to just "wing it" while drawing on their literacy in French. My usage of Hausa in this book attempts to follow Francophone conventions as well as Nigérien dialects of Hausa—there are several—most commonly spoken in Niamey. For example, the name given to me in a Nigérien village in 1988, is rendered as "Chaibou" in French-influenced Hausa, and as "Shaibu" in English-influenced Nigerian Hausa. I spell the Hausa word for heat as *zahi*, following the most common pronunciation heard in Niamey. Hausa dictionaries, which are typically based on the Kano, Nigeria, dialect, spell it as *zafi*, as it is pronounced there. Finally, I use typical names of people in Niamey as pseudonyms throughout the book to protect the privacy of participants.

## Overview of the Chapters

Chapter 1 traces the history of traditional medicine, Islamic medicine, and biomedicine in Niamey, highlighting links between medical pluralism and medical mistrust and the ways that these three medical sectors change, overlap, and influence each other. Chapter 2 focuses on a regional illness complex involving imbalances of "heat" and "cold." My examination reveals how medical pluralism and medical mistrust play out in relation to the most common health problems in Niamey. In Chapter 3, I argue that medical mistrust must be taken seriously. I argue that medical mistrust and trust can be absolute but seldom are. Instead, they coexist on a continuum. I center on the pervasiveness of medical mistrust in Niamey, identifying common factors across medical sectors that contribute to medical mistrust as well as specific reasons that Nigériens mistrust traditional medicine, Islamic medicine, and biomedicine. Chapter 4 builds on previous chapters. It features two extended case studies—one of a group of people and the other of single person—that illustrate the ways Nigériens navigate options within and between traditional, Islamic, and biomedical sectors both sequentially and simultaneously despite widespread mistrust of each sector. Chapter 5 examines the mistrust–trust continuum from the perspective of healers, detailing the overlapping and different strategies used by traditional, Islamic, and biomedical healers to overcome the medical mistrust of Nigériens. It emphasizes the importance of creative manipulations of the material culture of medicine to generate trust among patients. Chapter 6 offers an analysis of extreme, contextual medical mistrust by considering Nigérien perspectives on COVID-19. I explain why so many Nigériens doubt the very existence of the disease and are extremely wary about testing and vaccinations. The conclusion reviews the key theoretical and ethnographic contributions of the book, before suggesting that we can learn valuable lessons from the example of Niger that are applicable to medical mistrust in the U.S. and elsewhere.

## CHAPTER 1

# A Brief History of Medical Pluralism in Niamey, 1900–2024

## Introduction

Over time, Nigériens have absorbed, adapted, and "Nigérienized" traditional medicine, Islamic medicine, and biomedicine. One day a few years ago while hanging out in a streetside conversation group with old friends on a modestly busy street off the paved road network of Niamey, we observed four dyadic medical interactions occurring simultaneously in a very small space on the street and adjacent to it. A middle-aged man stopped his pushcart to sell one of two dozen or so varieties of traditional plant medicines to a woman customer. A young woman carrying plastic bottles with medicine for "heat" (*zahi* in Hausa, *weyno* in Zarma-Songhay) from a basin atop her head was asked to stop to sell some by a group of middle-aged men. A mobile vendor with a tower on his shoulder featuring about 30 pharmaceutical drugs lowered his tower and placed in the stool he was carrying over his shoulder so that a prospective customer could examine his products at eye level. All of this was transpiring virtually on the doorstep of an Islamic medicine shop—a 10-meter-square boutique constructed of painted sheet metal—where the pharmacist was consulting with a patient in the doorway.

It is unusual but not rare to see all these things happening at once in Niger. We were witnessing a microcosm of today's therapeutic pluralism in Niamey—and reflecting on it. The male traditional healer was selling plants to treat itching. The female traditional healer sold only medicine for "heat"— an untranslatable condition that is the most commonly treated illness in Niamey. The pharmaceutical vendor was likely selling a cold medication but may have been selling something for malaria. The Islamic pharmacist was

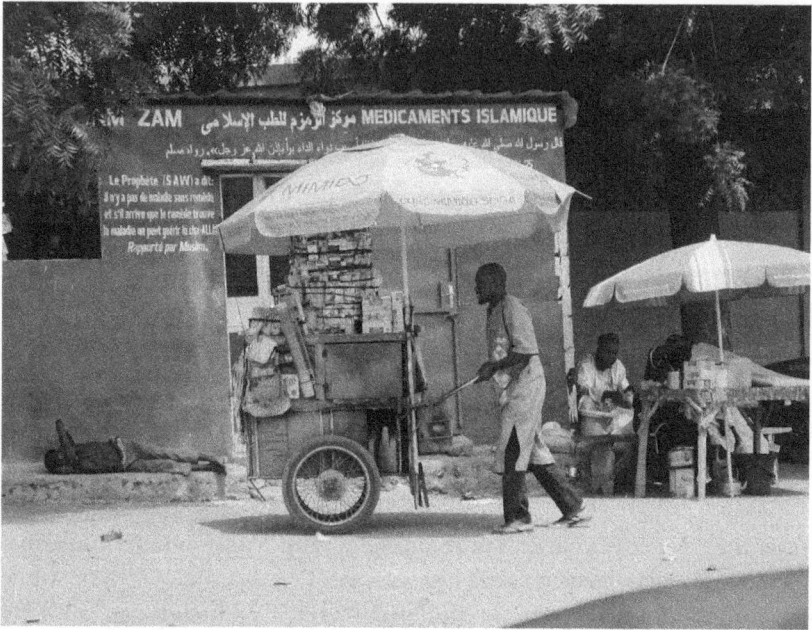

Figure 1.1. Itinerant pharmaceutic healer in front of an Islamic medicine shop.
Photo by author.

probably selling something to combat witchcraft, sorcery, or spirits because
boxed medicines designed for these purposes take up three-quarters of his
shelf space.

Each type of healer has something special to offer. Some traditional healers claim that they can cure all illnesses including cancer and HIV/AIDS
and that there is no need to visit Islamic pharmacists or biomedical facilities.
The women—mostly Nigérien but also many Beninoises and Togolaises—who
sell medicine for "heat" sell only this one product. It is widely perceived to
be efficacious in alleviating symptoms of this ubiquitous ailment for which
"there is no real cure" (Olivier de Sardan 1998, 194). The mobile vendors of
pharmaceuticals assert that they have medicines that can heal all illnesses
of natural, biological origin. While they do not purport to cure supernatural afflictions, they claim that they can treat some of the symptoms such as
headaches. Most Islamic pharmacists in Niamey sell *habatou saouda* (black
cumin seeds), which is said "to cure all ailments except death." Reflecting on

these grandiose assertions across street-level healers, Nigérien public health official Mariama Mounkaila sarcastically commented, "It is a wonder that everyone in Niamey does not live long, healthy lives and that healers are not fabulously wealthy!"

Understanding of contemporary medical pluralism in Niamey featuring three vibrant sectors—traditional, Islamic, and biomedical—requires some historical contextualization. The city and its therapeutic landscape have changed dramatically in the last 125 years. Diverse peoples have shaped Niamey's unique identity and character through time. For hundreds of years (and probably more) until the onset of French colonial rule at the turn of the 20th century, Niamey consisted of a collection of small fishing villages—Goudel, Saga, Lamordé, Bitinkidji, and Gamkalé—situated alongside the banks of the Niger River and inhabited by a few hundred Zarma, Songhay, Mawri, and Fulani peoples (Gado 1997, 9,14). The area surrounding Niamey was (and remains) primarily Zarma and Songhay country, with some interspersion of Fulani and Tuareg.

Nigériens used traditional therapies involving medicinal plants and spirits when they faced health problems in Niamey in 1900—as they had for countless generations—and this continued through the end of the colonial era in 1960 and until today. There were almost certainly a few Islamic healers in Niamey in 1900, but it is important to emphasize that at the time only a small minority of Nigériens were Muslims (Cooper 2019, 24; Fugelstad 1983, 116; Idrissa 2017, 64), even though Islam and Islamic medicine arrived in the region roughly 1,000 years ago. France gradually brought biomedical healthcare to Niger beginning around 1900—in 1922 there were only five doctors in the country (Fugelstad 1983, 116)—but it was reserved primarily for colonial administrators and the military, and Nigériens were largely denied access to it throughout the colonial era (Cooper 2019, 19–20). French colonial infrastructure was built on policies of inclusion and exclusion, and these had consequences for health. For example, the original treated, piped water network was limited to the Plateau neighborhood where the French lived and worked, while Nigériens relied on untreated well water or water from the Niger River (Keough and Youngstedt 2019, 26). Since independence, the piped water network has expanded, but even today about two-thirds of people in Niamey do not have running water at home. They rely on daily deliveries of water to their households provided by professional water carriers who use pushcarts containing eight to ten 20-liter containers of water that they have gathered at public standpipes, and on one-half-liter clear plastic bags of sachet water purchased from street vendors.

France chose Niamey as the colonial capital of Niger in 1926, and it continued to serve as the capital after Niger gained its independence in 1960. Much of its growth and diversity have been due to migration. Through the last 125 years of its history, first- and second-generation migrants have constituted a majority of the population. Waves of migrants from across Niger settled wherever they could find affordable lodging in Niamey such that by about 1980 (and ever since) the city has been residentially integrated by ethnicity, though it is segregated by class. Hausa migrants played a central role in the rapid growth of Niamey from a small city of 33,816—of whom only 3,600, or 12 percent, were Hausa in 1960 (Sidikou 1980; Bernus 1969, 35; Decalo 1989, 165)—to a bustling West African metropolis of two million residents today. The Hausa community grew to about the size of the Zarma community by about 1980 and the two have remained about equal in size up to the present. This constitutes a highly unusual transformation given that Niamey rests some 150 kilometers west of the westernmost boundaries of traditional Hausaland. Furthermore, people of dozens of West African ethnic groups, especially from Benin, Mali, Mauritania, Nigeria, Senegal, and Togo, also live in Niamey, and have brought some of their traditional medicine and medical practices with them. Today, Hausa and Zarma are the lingua francas of Niamey. French is also important in Niamey as Niger's official language, the primary language of media, and as a written language (for example, in medical packaging), but it is less widely spoken than Hausa and Zarma.

The mixing of people in Niamey offers people many opportunities to exchange ideas about health and healing and for a wide variety of forms of medicine to circulate. Today in Niamey, traditional, Islamic, and biomedical sectors are roughly equal in popularity. More than 90 percent of people in Niamey use traditional medicine at least occasionally, as my interviews indicate. Muslims became a majority in Niamey around 1960 (Idrissa 2017) and today 98 percent of residents identify as Muslim, leading to the rising credibility and use of Islamic medicine. Since independence, Nigériens in Niamey have gradually gained access to formal-sector public and private biomedical hospitals, clinics, and pharmacies, despite major setbacks when Niger took a neoliberal turn in the 1980s, 1990s, and 2000s by accepting structural adjustment programs and reducing public spending on health care.[1] The major turning point in terms of access to biomedicine began about 25 years ago with the commencement and proliferation of informal street vending of pharmaceutical drugs. The two developments were linked; that is, the neoliberal turn led to rising costs of medicines in the formal sector, making them unaffordable for many poor people, and this inspired entrepreneurs to seize an opportunity by entering the informal market to sell pharmaceutical drugs at far lower prices than those in formal-sector pharmacies.

Niamey is filled with laughter and joy, despite the severe poverty faced by many residents. Many Nigériens in Niamey find patience and strength through their humble devotion to Islam. They cherish their vibrant sociability and gracious hospitality, and deeply value extraordinary conversational virtuosity and knowledge. They deploy humor in complex transcendent, defensive, and self-critical ways, strive relentlessly to feel connected to the modern world at large, and perpetuate a sense of optimism for the future, despite the Islamic fatalism I referenced earlier. Niamey is a remarkably vibrant, lively, sociable place featuring a distinctive cosmopolitan, public, outdoor culture. The most common jobs—in trading, services, and manual work—take place outdoors. Most prayers are performed in open-air mosques and in sidewalk gatherings that sometimes expand to block off roads. Most men participate several hours daily in street-corner conversation groups. Women—carrying loads atop their heads and babies strapped to their backs—are constantly coming and going to markets, to work, or to visit family and friends. Children are ubiquitous in the streets—playing football games, laughing, and engaging in micro-commerce to support their families.

Niamey is more acutely and directly influenced by global trends, policies, and technologies than other places in Niger. Niamey clearly serves as Niger's most important "gateway to the global world" (Hansen 2008, 4). This includes access to new forms of traditional, Islamic, biomedical products of diverse provenance. Biomedical facilities are few and far between in rural Niger. If they have the means or a support network, rural Nigériens travel to Niamey to seek medical care, especially at Hôpital National de Niamey. Niamey also stands apart from the rest of the country due to its size and political and economic influence, and it is essential to Niger as it is intricately connected economically and through communication technology, transportation, kinship ties, and the circulation of medicines to even the most remote areas of the country.

Niamey is one of the world's fastest growing cities in one of the world's fastest growing, poorest, and youngest—the median age is 15 years—countries. Nigérien women have 7.6 children on average—the world's highest fertility rate (Cooper 2019, 1). By comparison, the fertility rate in the U.S. is 1.7 births per woman: Globally the fertility rate is 2.3 (World Bank 2023). It is also a place where people of all the country's ethnic groups live in roughly the same proportions as they do in the country as a whole. These include primarily Hausa, Zarma, Songhay, Mawri, Fulani, and Tuareg, and to a much lesser extent, Arab, Kanuri, Gourmantche, Tubu, Wogo, Korgo, Kourtey, and a host of others from West Africa, Lebanon, and elsewhere. Niamey is thus simultaneously the most and least representative place of Niger, and unlike other places in Niger that tend to be populated by one or a few ethnic groups. This also means that it is a place where a wide variety of groups bring their own understandings of healing, including variations of traditional medicine.

Niamey is characterized by *brassage*—a complex, fluid swirl of people, cultures, languages, and healing practices that has led in the past 20 years to the emergence of a new transethnic urban culture (Alidou 2005, 8). People in Niamey are exposed to a wide range of healing practices—traditional, Islamic, and biomedical—that derive from various ethnicities and regions. The exceptional amount of mixing—encouraged by the outdoor culture and residential neighborhoods that are generally not segregated by ethnicity—means that people can easily garner knowledge about an immense range of healing practices. This has led to a cosmopolitan culture of openness to diverse medical practices.

To make sense of the complexity and diversity of health and healing beliefs and practices in Niamey, I incorporate and adapt diverse perspectives from the vast literature on medical pluralism in Africa[2] and elsewhere.[3] Four themes are particularly important to my analysis. First, drawing from anthropologist Susan Rasmussen's (2001) *Healing in Community* and following the recent work of historian Jonathan Roberts (2021) in *Sharing the Burden of Sickness*, I argue that understanding medical pluralism requires *historical contextualization* that highlights the point and circumstances of the arrival of medical cultures and how they have changed over time. I also introduce the argument that medical mistrust is embedded in history, and that if we want to understand how it operates in medical sectors, we need to analyze how it has developed and shifted over time.

Second, I argue that it is important to *carefully define medical sectors* from multiple perspectives. I find sociologist David Baronov's (2008) approach articulated in *The African Transformation of Western Medicine* to be useful in this regard. He argues that medical systems consist of three main dimensions: empirical, interpretive, and conceptual. The empirical dimension involves behavior and the material culture of medicine and medical technologies. In Niger, this includes medical packaging and ways that medicines are displayed on medicine towers, pushcarts, and tables. The interpretive dimension considers medical systems as key symbolic-cultural expressions. Nigériens recognize that a stomachache may be caused by eating spoiled food, or by disrespecting one's parents. The conceptual dimension emphasizes that medical systems are expressions and forms of social power. As everywhere in the world, in Niamey, the healer–patient dyad is an asymmetrical power relationship that can almost inherently lead to some level of mistrust. This appeared during the initial months the COVID-19 pandemic, when government officials attempted to restrict people's movements and gatherings, and required masks, handwashing, vaccinations, and testing for certain categories of people. My interviews revealed that most people in Niamey chose their own medicines to treat COVID-19 or did absolutely nothing, based on the widespread idea that they were not threatened by it and that, further, it might be a conspiracy by the Nigérien state or the WHO. Baronov (2008, 25) argues that we must consider all three because "each sphere is distinct from yet inseparable from the other two." In sum, behaviors, thoughts, power, and resistance to power are intertwined.

Furthermore, in a classic anthropological approach, I emphasize emic perspectives; that is, local perspectives on medical pluralism. People in Niamey think about medical pluralism in diverse ways based on factors including social identity, age, gender, and occupation. Most notably, healers typically regard each sector as distinct, and they maintain practices specific to their sectors. Traditional healers sell only traditional medicines. Islamic healers sell only Islamic medicines. Mobile biomedicine vendors dispense only pharmaceuticals. Nevertheless, some healers cooperate and share information with healers of other sectors, some refer clients to healers of other sectors in particular situations, and some use medicines of all sectors in their own lives. In contrast, patients are less likely to regard each sector as separate. Many have medicines of all three systems in their home medicine collections at any time, and many use medicines and other therapies of each system sequentially or simultaneously. Indeed, Baronov (2008, 184) argues that "from the perspective of these persons, this is not a movement between discreet systems but between various therapeutic options within a single pluralistic-medical system."

Third, I examine and highlight *the link between medical pluralism and medical mistrust*. Both topics have been studied extensively, but few scholars have carefully considered the ways that they are connected. I argue that in Niger medical pluralism and medical mistrust must be studied together because neither can be fully understood without the other.

Fourth, I analyze the ways that traditional, Islamic, and biomedical *sectors change, overlap, and influence one another* while highlighting the *local and global mobility and circulation* of patients, healers, traders, medicines, and medical knowledge. The following overview of each medical sector touches on each of these four themes. I will also return to these at various places later in the book.

## Traditional Medicine in Niger

Given that hominids have lived in what is now Niger for several million years and given the conventional wisdom that healing was the first specialized "occupation," we can conclude that people living in the region have practiced forms of traditional medicine for a very long time. I emphasize that traditional healers and medicines are constantly changing and adapting—in recent times, partly in response to changes in and competition with Islamic medicine and biomedicine. I regard anything that Nigériens call "traditional medicine" as "traditional medicine" to differentiate it from other forms of medicine. I also use the term "traditional medicine" because it is the term used by Nigériens— *la médecine traditionelle* in French and *maganin gargajiya* in Hausa. The Hausa word *magani* means medicine, remedy and more broadly that which restores order. Other Nigérien languages have similar terms. For example, in Tamashek (the language of Tuareg people), *amagal* means medicine, protection, a solution to a problem, or anything that establishes balance and order (Rasmussen 2001, xxviii).

Nigérien traditional medicine, from an empirical perspective, customarily involves parent-child "inheritance," meaning that healers are born to other healers of either gender or both. Traditional healers must undergo extensive training—typically 20 years or more—before they can fully activate and hone their power to begin practicing on their own. To a lesser extent, traditional healers are trained in non-familial apprenticeships. Until recently these apprenticeships in Niger almost always took place within ethnic groups, but as my interviews indicate, increasing numbers of would-be healers are learning their craft from healers outside of their ethnic groups. This is an important development that is leading to new forms of medical pluralism. The emerging practice of training taking place across families and ethnic groups also contributes to contemporary mistrust of traditional medicine among Nigériens because they tend to trust healers with inborn, natural power over those without it. Nigérien traditional medicine also includes a scientific approach featuring empirical observation and trial-and-error testing. (Falen [2018] refers to traditional healing in Southern Benin as "African science" because it also involves these practices.) Nigérien traditional medicine is all about the quest for knowledge of esoteric secrets and power: "power to cure sickness, increase bodily strength, eliminate vulnerability, gain popularity, increase sexual potency or attractiveness [and fertility], obtain financial success, eliminate a rival" (Wall 1988, 294) or to achieve other goals.

Nigérien traditional medicine consists of two branches that are sometimes intertwined: medicines and spirit therapies. Nigériens in Niamey collectively recognize a vast pharmacopeia of more than 1,000 plants, trees, and shrubs, including their roots, bark, leaves, flowers, twigs, and seeds. They also use minerals, stones, clay, insects, animal parts and droppings, and honey as medicines. These are administered in a wide range of ways, including via food or liquid, creams, incense, and injection. Nigérien traditional medicine also involves surgeries, including uvulectomies,[4] bloodletting,[5] male circumcision,[6] and female cutting[7]. These traditional surgeries, except for female cutting, are performed by male "barber-surgeons" (wanzamai in Hausa), who also shave men's heads and faces. The second branch involves working with spirits in various ways—sometimes to exorcise them but more often to communicate with them (for example, to learn healing secrets) or to placate them with music, perfume, and animal sacrifice during spirit possession ceremonies. A wide range of spirits animate Nigérien worlds, including unnamed, everyday ones that are everywhere; named ones with known personalities and tastes that reside in particular places but can also travel great distances instantaneously; ones that possess human hosts only when summoned; and ones that can possess human hosts against their will either individually or in large groups, as happened with whole classrooms of schoolgirls (Casey 2021, Masquelier 2020).

Due to the recent rise of reformist Salafist Islam in Niamey, spirit possession ceremonies have been suppressed and are now rare in Niamey. The Salafi movement advocates a return to the authentic Islam practiced by the Prophet Muhammad and early generations of Muslims, and stresses that placating spirits is contrary to Islam. According to linguistic anthropologist/ethnomusicologist Brian Nowak (2019), 20 years ago about 20 possession troupes were active in Niamey whereas today there are only four. These troupes are teams

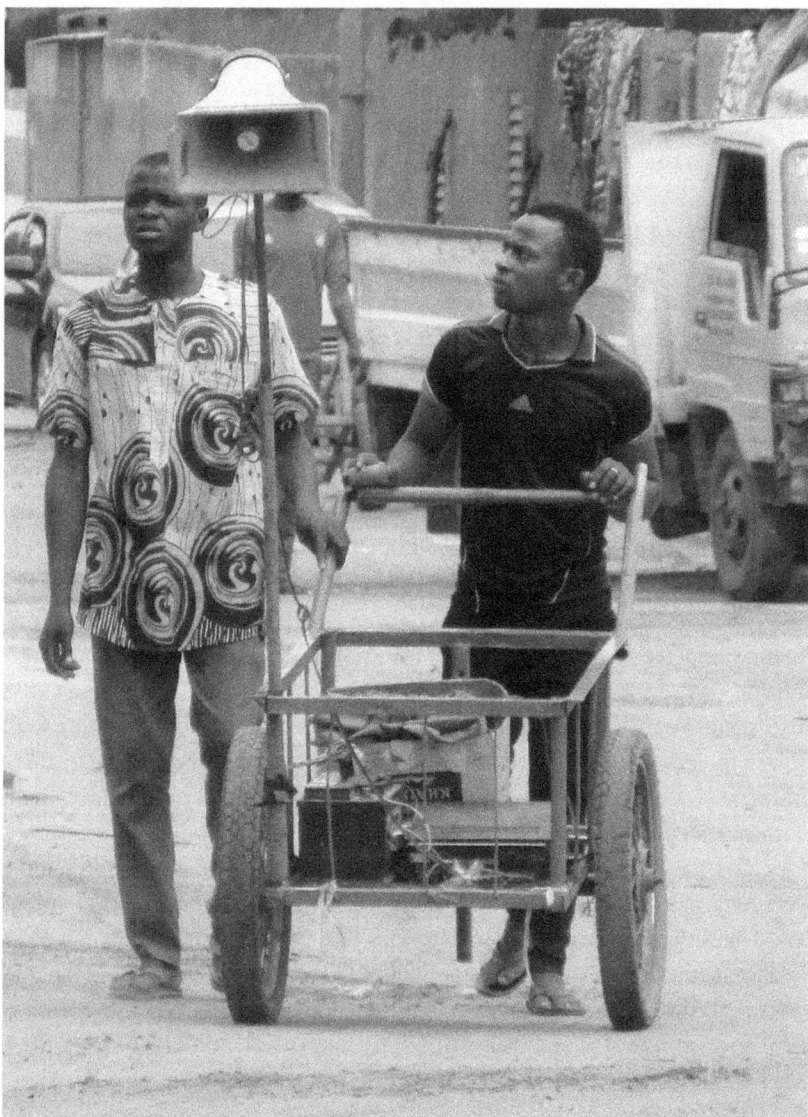

Figure 1.2. Traditional healers with plant medicines on pushcart. Photo by author.

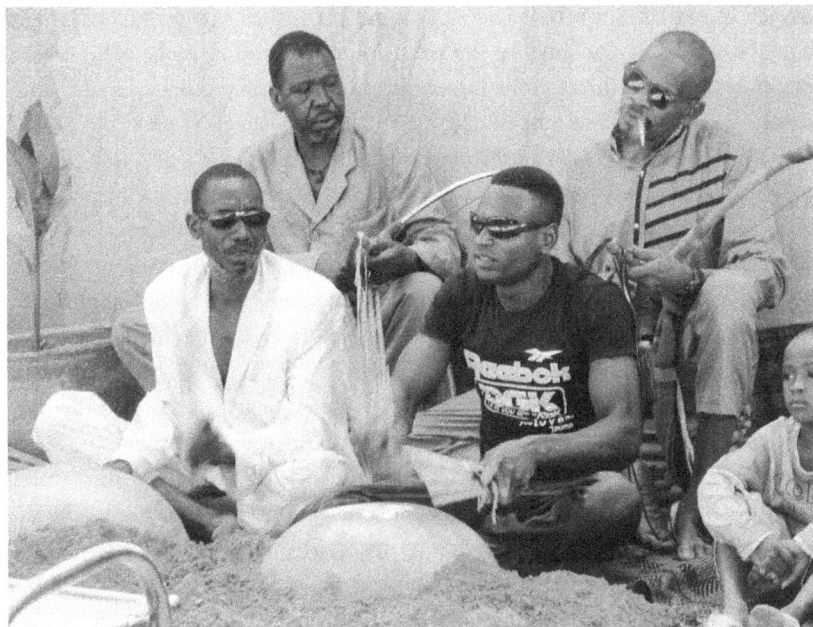

Figure 1.3. *Bori* musical group praising spirits. Photo by author.

of several men that include one-stringed violinists, calabash drummers, and praise-singers who know the specific songs that specific spirits like. This music is intended to attract and flatter spirits and encourage them to possess afflicted people in order to diagnose their problems and alleviate them. Some Nigériens leave Niamey to return to their rural home regions for these healing rituals. They typically share this experience only with their closest family, keeping their therapeutic regimens compartmentalized (Youngstedt 2013).

Nigérien traditional medicine interprets health and illness holistically as it recognizes natural, supernatural, and socio-emotional etiologies and considers them as overlapping. For this reason, Baronov (2008) refers to African traditional medicine as "African pluralist medicine." Imbalance or disruption in the social world and one's place it may also lead to illness directly or indirectly. Conflict, jealousy, anxiety, disrespect, and malicious gossip may lead to physical illness, and victims of disrespect may use sorcery to attack people who have slighted them. "Illnesses of Allah" are caused by inanimate, unconscious forces in the physical environment, what can be labeled "natural causes." This includes consuming unclean or tainted food or water;

overeating sweet, sour, bitter, or salty foods; exposure to too much heat and cold. "Illnesses of evil" involve the intrusion of conscious, malevolent power, either by spirits or through the human agency of sorcery and witchcraft. Spirits can serve as explanations for almost any illness, especially any long-lasting enfeebling pathological conditions such as migraines, epilepsy, hunchback, paralysis, blindness, dementia, deafness, and leprosy. The traditional religions of Niger center on efforts to maintain harmony and balance with the spirit world through spirit possession and other forms of communication such as music. For example, the *Bori* religion of the Hausa includes hundreds of named spirits and many of them are thought to cause specific illnesses.

Echoing the famous work of E. E. Evans-Pritchard (1937) on the Azande of Sudan, most Nigérien cultures regard witchcraft and sorcery as distinct, while recognizing that there can be overlap between them. Witches of Niger wield inherent evil power, typically acquired through their mothers' milk. In Niger, they are known to eat the souls of people, causing them to waste away and die if their souls are not returned through the aid of specialists (Schmoll 1993). Some witch-detecting techniques are practiced in Niger, but witchcraft accusations are rare—few are identified by name—in sharp contrast with neighboring Benin (Falen 2018) and Cameroon (Geschiere 1997; Geshiere and Fisiy 1994). Sorcery involves consciously learned techniques of using medicine for evil purposes as well as for good ones. Although witchcraft accusations are rare, many Nigériens think that witches inflict pain and suffering on their enemies; similarly, sorcery is often named as a possible cause of illnesses. Both witches and sorcerers draw on techniques of traditional medicine and may work as healers themselves. All of this contributes to doubt and fear about traditional medicine sellers. In the minds of some Nigériens, since traditional healers have the power to alleviate complex problems they may also be able to use these powers to harm people.[8]

Another distinctive feature of Nigérien traditional medicine is its receptive, pragmatic attitude toward other medical concepts and practices, including various forms of West African medicine, Islamic medicine, and biomedicine. This parallels the ways that Nigériens (and Africans in general) think about and indigenize foreign ideas in contrast with the attitude of foreigners about Nigérien ideas. In the last century, *Bori*, the traditional Hausa religion, incorporated French soldier spirits (Masquelier 2001, 162), Muslim spirits (Masquelier 2001, 222), a British anthropologist (Last 2011, 219), and Bollywood spirits (Casey 2021, 132). Those who practice traditional religions in Niger are not ostracized in traditional religious communities when they become Muslims or Christians. This contrasts with Muslims in Niger who are denigrated when they practice traditional local religions, especially anything involving appeasing spirits in any way. For many Muslims in Niger, worst of all is mixing Islam with "pagan" traditional religions, which is even worse than being a "pure pagan." However, mixing across religions occurs across many contexts. For example, Rasmussen (2001, 90) documented that among the Tuareg, diviners sometimes combine Qur'anic and non-Qur'anic techniques, and that to garner respect in the community, even traditional, non-Qur'anic healers should be seen as good Muslims who pray and generously give alms. Some healers use both Qur'anic texts and traditional magical powders in making protective amulets, as I have observed among Hausa and Zarma.

Traditional healers in Niger take pride in their craft and consider healing as fulfilling a social obligation to their communities. Traditional healing services have long been commodified in Niger, but many healers do not charge set fees. Rather, they charge patients based on their means or allow patients to determine how much to pay. Some healers in Niamey develop long-term—even lifelong—relationships with patients and families, while many others have only one-time encounters with patients. Most healer–patient relationships fall in between these extremes. Many Nigériens in Niamey have a preferred "go-to" traditional healer, but none of the people I interviewed indicated that they visit only one traditional healer.

Today it is difficult to distinguish traditional medicine practices of the country's various ethnic groups. Until 20 to 40 years ago, it made some sense to refer to the ethnomedicine of specific ethnic groups in Niger—Hausa medicine, Zarma medicine, and so on. Even so, 36 years ago in *Hausa Medicine: Illness and Well-Being in a West African Culture*, anthropologist and biomedical doctor L. Lewis Wall (1988, 324) concluded that "medical knowledge is transmitted within very narrow family traditions, or to apprentice adepts, and there is no clearly defined 'Hausa medical tradition' standardized, taught, and generally accepted throughout Hausaland—only a range of ideas and accepted therapies that exist in many different forms in many different areas." Similarly, Rasmussen (2001, 59) argued that there is no monolithic healing system with unitary principles and practices among the Tuareg, but rather "multiple, potential, and emergent healing communities." Historian Jonathan Roberts (2021, 8) argues that "no longer can we think of Africans as possessing indigenous ethnomedicines; the healing landscape of the continent has been changing for so long that it is now a place with clusters of therapeutic regimes competing in each region." These clusters of therapeutic regimes are adapted to clusters of locally recognized health concepts and illnesses. A prime example of this is an illness complex centered around the imbalance between "heat" and "cold" involving both diverse internal symptoms and external visible symptoms, and a wide variety of therapies to treat them.

Nigériens have always shared medicine and therapies across ethnic lines—what Baronov (2008) calls "African syncretic medicine"—and this process is accelerating especially in the transethnic urban culture of Niamey. Traditional healers in Niamey have begun sharing knowledge and medicines across ethnic lines in a focused, deliberate way particularly through the establishment of the l'Association des Tradi-Practiciens du Niger (ATPN) in 1995, in contrast with the longstanding practice of passing the art and science of traditional healing through narrow family lines. This group has become vital in efforts to defend and promote traditional healing.

Traditional healers in Niamey continuously change and adapt to a pluralistic medical environment in many other ways. Most traditional healers today are Muslims who have also come to respect the power of biomedicine to treat illnesses of natural causes, especially through technologies and procedures such as x-rays and surgery. Some use Islamic medicine and biomedicines in particular circumstances. They have learned to identify and treat relatively newly emerging problems in Niamey, such as obesity, diabetes, and hypertension that are the result of the transition from local foods (millet, sorghum, cowpeas, vegetables) and active lifestyles to processed "prestige" foods (polished rice and wheat, Maggi cubes, sugar, pasta) and sedentary lifestyles (Cooper 2019, 228). Furthermore, traditional healers are embracing biomedical marketing strategies such as packaging their medicines and advertising through social media. These varied approaches illustrate the ways in which medical sectors overlap and demonstrate that traditional healers strategically adopt and adapt new healing practices and technologies.

The provenance of traditional medicines is diverse. Some traditional healers are experts in collecting plants and other medicine, which requires deep ecological knowledge and arduous work involving travel deep into the bush to climb rocky outcroppings and trees and dig roots in hard Sahelian soils. Other healers sell what their connections have collected, especially those in cities such as Niamey where they have limited or no direct access to the bush to collect medicines themselves. Furthermore, people regularly bring traditional medicine from neighboring countries to Niamey. Other traditional medicines have arrived recently in Niamey from further afield, such India and China, some of which are now being cultivated in Niger. For example, a team of entrepreneurs began cultivating and marketing artemisia in Niger in 2018 after receiving training in Benin provided by La Maison de l'Artemisia, an international network active in 28 countries that promotes the plant for the prevention and treatment of malaria. Two types are being grown in Niger today: "*Artemisia annua* . . . an herbaceous plant that has been used for 2000 years in Traditional Chinese Medicine to prevent and treat intermittent fevers (malaria) and other parasitic diseases . . . [and] . . . *Artemisia afra* . . . a perennial bush native to Southeast Africa, used by Traditional Medicine practitioners for centuries to prevent and cure malaria and other parasitic diseases" (La Maison de l'Artemisia 2021)

My brief overview has emphasized that traditional medicine in Niger retains some broad core principles but simultaneously is dynamic as healers continuously adapt to new circumstances. Traditional medicine in Niger emphasizes holism and the connections between physical, spiritual, and socio-emotional health and well-being as well as the importance of balancing "heat" and "cold" across all dimensions of life. Pragmatism and syncretism are important hallmarks of traditional medicine in Niger. Traditional healers share knowledge and medicines across ethnicities, and this process is accelerating. Furthermore, traditional medicine does not exist in a vacuum in Niger; it shares the therapeutic landscape with Islamic medicine and biomedicine. Over time, Islamic and biomedical spokesmen and healers have worked hard to discredit traditional medicine. Traditional healers have responded creatively, emphasizing pride in local cultural heritage while also learning and adapting knowledge and practices of Islamic medicine and biomedicine. Almost everyone in Niamey—more than 90 percent of the people that I interviewed—uses traditional medicines and therapies, though most people also use Islamic medicine and biomedicine. In short, the traditional medical sector flourishes in Niamey and throughout Niger because it remains relevant to the ways that millions of Nigériens think about health and well-being.

## Islamic Medicine in Niger

Islam and Islamic medicine arrived in the Niamey region about 1,000 years ago, as previously mentioned. Nigérien acceptance of the culture of Islam was a long, slow process. Islam arrived in the region largely through itinerant traders, but later many Nigériens were enslaved by Arab Muslims and forcibly transported to North Africa. This contributed to mistrust of Islam, Islamic medicine, and Muslims (Abdalla 1999, 179). Thus, mistrust is embedded in history. In contrast, part of the way that Islam gained ground in the region over time was by offering a novel medical system that "could apparently bring about victories, defend cities, assure rain, protect property, and ward off calamity and misfortune" (Abdalla 1992, 193). Today, mistrust of Islamic medicine is gendered in that Nigérien women are much more mistrustful of Islamic medicine than men are (Cooper 2019, 56, 60–61). Furthermore, Nigériens tend to be highly skeptical regarding new, recently arriving, imported Islamic medicines.

Abdalla (1992) sketches the *longue durée* of the history of Islam in Hausaland as consisting of three sometimes overlapping stages: compartmentalization, syncretism, reform. (Parallel processes took place among neighboring ethnic groups.) *Compartmentalization* refers to a relatively short period during which Islam and local religions were practiced separately. *Syncretism* refers to a long "period of gradual but slow acculturation and conversion characterized by mixing of Islamic and non-Islamic beliefs and practices . . . which manifested itself in the medical field" (Abdalla 1992, 192, 194). At some point in history, for example, healers began making protective amulets that included both traditional magic plant powders and Qur'anic passages written on folded pieces of paper. This was punctuated by periods of *reform* when leaders sought to purge Islam of local, non-Islamic practices, such as the Fulani jihad led by Usman dan Fodio in 1804 that resulted in the creation of the Sokoto Caliphate. Today Niger is in the midst of another reform movement with the rise of Salafist conservatism over the last two decades, sponsored and influenced by clerics in Saudi Arabia and Northern Nigeria (Idrissa 2017; Moussa 2023, 57). This development, I suggest, has amplified the importance of Islamic medicine in Niger, as I will detail below.

The spread of Islam in Niger impacted people's health in a variety of ways. Many Islamic ideas and practices regarding health have been beneficial to Nigériens, such as abstinence from alcohol, ritual ablutions five times daily, and various food practices, among others. In contrast, historian Barbara Cooper (2019, 229) carefully documented how the rapid rise in the number and percentage of Muslims in Niger in the late colonial period and ever since led to an important change in sexuality in marriage, namely a significant shortening of birth spacing. In Niger and the Sahel more generally, up until roughly the 1970s, the norm was for women to abstain from sex with their husbands for two years while they nursed their babies; however, "The widespread adoption of Muslim identity had by the 1980s nullified the moral force behind conjugal abstinence while nursing. Women no longer had the means to counter the newer [Islamic] pattern of resumption of conjugal relations after only forty days" (Cooper 2019, 230). Then, by the 2010s, Cooper (2019, 231) found that "most Muslim women . . . in Niamey had no collective memory of these earlier patterns of nursing and sexual restraint in marriage." The consequences of this change are unsurprising: "These new conditions imperiled the health of small children, and they also increased maternal mortality" (Cooper 2019, 231). Even though many women of Niger are not explicitly aware of how the relatively recent rise of Islam has impacted their experience of pregnancy and childbirth, for various reasons Nigérien women avoid Islamic medicine in general. Cooper (2019, 60–61) concludes "Islamic medicine has had surprisingly little purchase on the practices of women throughout Hausa-speaking regions, regardless of their degree of commitment to the orthodoxy of various reformists . . . [women] . . . hold tightly to [traditional] practices they find meaningful." This is particularly the case regarding the health outcome that Nigérien women fear most, infertility.

Scholars have had difficulty defining "Islamic medicine" not only because of differing disciplinary perspectives but more importantly because Islamic medicine has continuously changed, absorbed medical concepts of various cultures (for example, Greek humoral ideas), and has been contested within Muslim communities. Abdalla (1992, 178) argues that "neither in theory nor in practice was the medical experience of Muslims truly or exclusively Islamic. The Qur'an, whose word for Muslims is final in all other aspects of life, has little to say about medicine or healing." Feierman and Janzen (1992, 21), drawing from Abdalla (1992, 177–79), thus define Islamic medicine as "the medicine of Islamdom . . . encompassing all the diverse conceptions and practices of the Islamic world, regardless of whether the particular practices had Islamic theological roots" (Feierman and Janzen 1992, 21). I find this expansive, inclusive definition useful for approaching Niamey, particularly given continuous arrival of new Islamic medicines of diverse provenance that have led to debates about what constitutes "Islamic medicine" and the recent rise and proliferation of specialists in who refer to themselves as "Islamic pharmacists."

Islamic medicine in Niger, from an empirical perspective, involves faith and specialized knowledge of the Qur'an and the Hadiths—the traditions of the Prophet Muhammad. It has never been uniform in Niger, and is changing rapidly and increasingly contested—as is Islam in general in Niamey. It includes wide range of therapies such as prayer, plant medicine, diet (halal, fasting, honey as a "miracle food"), holy water (especially from the Zam Zam well of Mecca), vegetal chalk used in Qur'anic slates, and protective amulets consisting of folded pieces of paper with Qur'anic passages sewn into leather pouches. Islamic medicine in Niamey also includes esoteric practices known only to a few specialists such as divination, numerology, and spirit exorcism.

The core metaphysical foundation of Islamic medicine in Niger (and really, all medicine in Niger at this point) is that everything that happens is a result of Allah's will, including illness and recovery. For each illness, Allah has ordained a remedy. However, as Rasmussen (2001, xxx) points out, it is also the case that "for every remedy, there is also a danger, and remedies may become polluted, even poisonous." Subordinate to Allah is a body of sentient but capricious beings with lesser but still substantial powers including jinn (spirits) as well as witches and sorcerers. The Qur'an makes many references to jinn, as "bodiless beings made of smokeless fire who can shape-shift and move across space at great speed" (Masquelier 2019b, 187). In contrast, many Islamic scholars in Niamey teach that witches and sorcerers do not exist, that they are merely "African superstition." Masquelier (2019b) emphasizes that Muslims in Niger regard spirits very differently from those who adhere to traditional local beliefs and practices. Muslims regard spirits as inherently evil servants of Satan that must be exorcised when they possess human hosts. This is achieved through various techniques that forcefully expel spirits from the body such as the inhalation of noxious smoke of particular kinds of incense and the ingestion of various kinds of purgatives.

Traditionalists think of spirits as neither wholly evil nor wholly good. "Spirit devotees communicate with spirits to channel their powers productively" (Masqueler 2019b, 178), and view spirits as entities that can be negotiated with and placated in many cases. In other cases, traditional healers work to exorcise spirits that are harming possessed individuals. Some traditional healers and patients believe that Muslim techniques of handling spirits will never work, that they will only increase the anger of spirits and the danger to humans. This is another example of contextualized mistrust of Islamic therapeutics. That is, drawing from interview and focus group conversations, some Nigériens who trust Islamic medicine for treating many illnesses mistrust the ways Islamic healers deal with spirits. Occasionally, Islamic and traditional specialists work together to exorcise spirits (Casey 2021, Masquelier 2020). Islamic healers and patients grapple with a cosmic complexity wherein all illness and death are ultimately attributed to Allah, but Allah has provided remedies for all illnesses. Knowledge of these remedies requires intensive, life-long study of the Qur'an, and the sharing of medical secrets among specialists.

Islamic scholars and assorted healers feel that they are following Allah's will to protect their communities. They nevertheless accept renumeration for their services in cash or in kind. Furthermore, Islamic medicine in Niamey has become increasingly commodified in last decade or so with the rise and proliferation of healers calling themselves "Islamic pharmacists." This is an example of how Islamic medicine and healers continuously change and adapt. In recent years Islamic medicine healers, scholars, and vendors in Niamey have creatively used new marketing strategies and modern technology to disseminate information and to sell their products. Parallel to traditional medicine, most Islamic medicine was dispensed with scrap paper until 20 or so years ago but is now increasingly sold in labeled packages, including local medicines and especially imported medicines. In recent years, a wide variety of boxed medicines manufactured in Northern Nigeria (especially Kano) to combat witchcraft, sorcery, and spirits have arrived on the streets and in the Islamic pharmacies of Niamey. Whereas the marketing of these new products can be seen as part of the ongoing efforts among Islamic healers to gain the trust of clients, Nigériens generally view these new medicines with suspicion and mistrust. One of the reasons for this skepticism is that many Nigériens have been influenced by the sermons of certain Islamic leaders in Niger who preach that witches and sorcerers do not exist—as seen in the story of Mariama's husband, Abdourahmane, that opened the book.

The provenance of Islamic medicines in Niamey, especially the packaged varieties, is primarily foreign. Islamic medicines in Niamey are imported primarily from Saudi Arabia, Nigeria, Tunisia, India, and Morocco in that order, as I learned through interviews with Islamic pharmacists and by study-ing packaging labels. Though less common, others were made in Indonesia, Egypt, and Burkina Faso. The boxed medicines made in Nigeria feature vivid color images of witches, zombies, and demons that clearly borrow liberally from global popular culture and the horror film industry. Some Nigériens wonder what makes this "Islamic medicine." To promote their credibility, labels on Islamic medicine sold in Niamey almost always include Arabic let-tering, the name of the Islamic pharmacist who made it or supervised its production, and highlight that the contents are all natural and plant-based. Religion, in a sense, has become a business. Furthermore, Islamic medicine specialists now use social media as well as television and radio programs to reach ever-expanding audiences.

In sum, Nigériens have used Islamic medicine, broadly defined, for hundreds of years, but it is only recently that it has gained prominence. The acceptance and embracing of Islam and Islamic medicine in Niger was slowed to some degree by the trans-Saharan slave trade and its association with Arab Muslims as well as strong adherence to local religions, cosmologies, and medicines. Islamic medicine and traditional medicine have coexisted and influenced each other for so long in Niger that is some cases they are indistinguishable (cf. Sams 2017, 1110). The adoption of Islamic health and cultural practices had both positive and negative impacts on Nigériens' health. Today, about 98 percent of Nigériens identify as Muslim. Almost all Nigériens observe the core Islamic practices of five-times daily prayers and fasting during the month of Ramadan, which are regarded as morally, socially, and physically therapeutic. Beyond this, the degree to which Nigériens specifically seek out "Islamic medicine" varies considerably from many who rarely do so to others whose first choice when ill is Islamic medicine. As one of the people that Sams (2017, 1112) interviewed put it in reference to Islamic medicines from Saudi Arabia, "These are made for Muslims. By Muslims for Muslims. . ." Islamic medicine is gendered in Niger: most healers and patients are men. Nigérien women tend to mistrust Islamic healers or regard Islamic medicine as not useful for women. Ideas about proper Islamic belief and practice and medicine have been shifting rapidly and are increasingly contested in Niger, especially in the last 25 years. Until the late 1990s, almost all Islamic medicine used in Niger was made in Niger and dispensed or sold discreetly by marabouts or vendors outside of major mosques—what can aptly be called "traditional Islamic medicine of Niger." (Marabouts, a term used across North and West Africa, refers to Muslim holy men known for their healing powers.) Today, a considerable portion of Islamic medicine available in Niamey is industrially packaged and imported from a variety of countries and is increasingly being sold by men identifying as "Islamic pharmacists."

## Biomedicine in Niger

Biomedicine is the latest arrival to the therapeutic landscape in Niamey, as it first appeared there in the early 20th century. As such, it was associated with France's brutal conquest (Lemkin 2020), the colonial regime, racism, and exclusion—and still is to some extent. Nigériens were mostly denied access to biomedicine during the colonial era. French colonial rule had decidedly negative impacts on the health of Nigériens, as it led military conscription, forced labor, damaged ecosystems, and regular famines. Biomedicine's link to an alien and hostile culture meant that accepting it and adapting it to local needs was a long, slow, and still ongoing process. Biomedicine's initial impact in Niger was minimal for another reason. Unlike many colonies in Africa, where there was a significant Christian missionary presence that built hospitals and clinics, Niger never had many Christian missionaries. Since 1924, only the Sudan Interior Mission—an evangelical Christian organization led mostly by Americans—has worked directly in health care in Niger, especially with the operation of its hospital for 75 years in Galmi, a small town in south-central Niger (Cooper 2006, 10). Cooper (2006, 318) explains that "Although Nigériens looked on early colonial medical facilities, which were often staffed with military doctors, with mistrust and skepticism, they received the mission's medical work with great enthusiasm very quicky." Nigériens use the terms "modern medicine" (*médecine moderne* in French and *maganin zamani* in Hausa) and "hospital medicine" (*maganin asbiti* in Hausa) to describe "biomedicine." I will use these terms interchangeably.

Biomedicine, in terms of empiricism, involves specialized, uniform training and knowledge in applied biochemistry, complex technology, scientific rigor, and peer review. As an interpretive endeavor, biomedicine emphasizes strict adherence to principles of scientific objectivity. It attributes health and illness only to natural, biological causes. At a conceptual level, biomedicine is a form of social power, involving the commodification of medical services and medicine, and the concentration of power among biomedical corporations, institutions, and practitioners. In the minds of Nigériens, it is linked to the Nigérien state and to global institutions such as the WHO—and their public health policies.

Niamey's biomedical infrastructure includes two branches that are essentially separate in the view of many Nigériens: a formal sector and an informal sector. Even though both sectors dispense biomedical pharmaceutical drugs, Nigériens typically regard them as distinct medical systems due to significant differences with respect to the social distance between healers and patients, cost, and convenience. In contrast with formal-sector biomedical workers who often are condescending toward and sometimes will use only French with patients (even when they know their patients speak little French), street vendors typically treat clients with respect and speak with them in Nigérien languages.[9]

The formal sector includes public and private hospitals, clinics, and pharmacies. These formal-sector biomedical institutions use, prescribe, and sell medicines manufactured primarily in France and Germany. Niger has the lowest density of biomedical professional workers in the world. As medical anthropologists Kelley Sams and Tabitha Hrynick (2020, 6) report, "For a population of 23.3 million, the country's civil servants in public health care included only 757 medical doctors, 4,157 nurses and 697 midwives in 2016, mainly posted in urban areas . . . Over half of Niger's doctors live in Niamey (the capital city), while only 6% of the overall population does." (To put this into comparative perspective, there are 260 physicians per 100,000 people in the U.S., while there are only 2 physicians per 100,000 people in Niger. Furthermore, physicians in the U.S. are far more likely to have access to the equipment and medicines to do their work than their counterparts in Niger.) Niamey hosts 21 pharmacies, 20 clinics, and 12 hospitals, including two major hospitals—Hôpital National de Lamordé and Hôpital National de Niamey.

Even though the biomedical infrastructure of Niamey is far more extensive than it is in Niger as a whole, it suffers from a chronic lack of resources and overworked and corrupt staff. Many negative experiences in hospitals—and the widespread circulation of stories about them—contribute significantly to the widespread mistrust of biomedicine in Niger, especially of the public sector. The private sector of biomedicine has expanded significantly over the past 30 years largely as a result of global neoliberal policies that pushed Niger toward privatization of all essential services. The private sector offers better care than the public sector, but it is not affordable to the masses. When Niamey's truly wealthy fall ill, they do not trust these facilities; instead, they simply hop on airplanes to visit hospitals in France.

One major change over time is that formal-sector biomedical facilities in postcolonial times are now staffed primarily by Nigériens, especially after the medical school at Université Abdou Moumouni was established in 1974. Most are Muslims who also have some understanding of local traditional concepts of health and illness. Nigérien biomedical professionals express a range of stances regarding traditional medicine. Some, following "the company line," belittle and disparage traditional healing and healers. Others refer patients to traditional healers, for example for spirit afflictions, and many use traditional medicine themselves. Thus, many biomedical specialists in Niger are deeply implicated in medical pluralism in their professional practices and personal health choices.

Another even more significant change in the biomedical sector involved the rise of the informal street vending of pharmaceutical drugs 25 years ago and its proliferation ever since, especially in the last decade. Medical anthropologist Carine Baxerres (2001) argued that pharmaceutical regulations in formerly French colonies in West Africa are modeled after France where medications—including ibuprofen—can be sold only in formal-sector pharmacies, which led to the proliferation of informal itinerant vendors, a form of resistance or "globalization from below." Because they typically offer generic pharmaceuticals and offer dosing flexibility—they regularly sell one pill at a time—mobile vendors sell their drugs for a small fraction of the prices demanded by formal-sector pharmacies that primarily sell name-brand pharmaceuticals and sell only full courses of treatment or full bottles or boxes of medicine. Nigériens also appreciate that they can negotiate prices and negotiate or even determine their therapies with informal pharmaceutical vendors, just as they can with traditional and Islamic healers, in sharp contrast with their interactions with biomedical personnel. The pharmaceutical medicines sold on the streets of Niamey are manufactured primarily in the Global South. Most of the drugs sold by mobile vendors are generics produced especially in India, but also in China, Indonesia, Egypt, Morocco, Kenya, Ghana, and Nigeria. Many of the drugs now have names in local languages, and some of the drugs are prescribed and/or used in ways that were not intended by manufacturers. Many Nigériens use various cold medicines for energy because they include caffeine, not for treating colds. Others use antibiotics for treating any fever even when the cause is unknown. These processes illustrate the broader "African transformation of biomedicine" and the rise of African biomedicine identified by Baronov (2008).

Nigériens were mostly denied access to biomedicine during the colonial era, and accessing biomedicine remains difficult today primarily due to its cost and, for the 75 percent of Nigériens who live in rural areas, long distances to travel from their homes to hospitals or clinics. Mistrust of biomedicine lingers among many Nigériens, especially regarding public health facilities and state-mandated public health policies. Two important developments over the past 25 years or so have radically transformed the biomedical sector in Niamey. Biomedical facilities in Niamey are increasingly staffed by Nigériens, and this has played a role in the growth in trust of biomedicine. Many Nigériens trust hospital medicine today for treating their most serious illnesses, or at least mistrust it less than traditional and Islamic medicine in some cases. The parking lot and entrance to the Hôpital National de Niamey buzzes with activity and taxis coming and going day and night. The rise of informal street vending of pharmaceutical drugs is an even more significant change, diverting what were formerly, and still are legally, "enclaved commodities" (Appadurai 1986, 24), and making them available for general exchange.

## Further Insights on Medical Pluralism in Niamey

None of the three medical sectors is dominant or even fully controls a corner of the Niamey health-care market. Biomedicine has gained importance in recent years, especially in the informal sector, but it has not supplanted traditional and Islamic medicine. Indeed, all three sectors are expanding and flourishing. As long as Nigériens continue to view health and illness as holistically involving the interplay of natural, supernatural, and social factors, there will always be room for traditional and Islamic medicine.

Healers in Niamey compete for clients within and between medical sectors. They do so in two primary ways. First, traditional, Islamic and biomedical healers tout their own virtues with appeals to cultural heritage, faith, and modernity, respectively. Second, healers of specific sectors seek to discredit the principles, practices, and healers of different sectors. They sometimes also do so vis-à-vis healers within their own sectors. These are major factors that contribute to medical mistrust in Niamey and lead many Nigériens to conclude that they cannot all be right. In a context of pervasive doubt and skepticism, patients "shop their sickness around" a wide range of options—to borrow Roberts's phrase (2021, 10). Sometimes it is not about finding a healer or therapy one fully trusts, but about finding someone or something one mistrusts the least among accessible and affordable choices.

Still other issues contribute to the pluralistic therapeutic scene in Niamey. In Nigérien medical sectors, the same illnesses can have different symptoms; and similar symptoms can be due to vastly different illnesses. Natural ailments may present themselves in ways that are indistinguishable from problems caused by spirits. A stomachache can be caused by eating spoiled food or by a spirit attack. Furthermore, social disruption—such as jealousy, disputes, or disrespecting one's parents—can also lead to physical ailments. This presents challenges for making diagnoses and is part of the reason that multiple healing sectors flourish in Niamey. In many cases, therapies are used to make diagnoses within and between medical sectors. For example, ailments that do not respond to biomedical treatment are presumed to be caused by supernatural forces.

Drawing from anthropologist Arjun Appadurai's (1986) influential work on "the social life of things," medical anthropologists Susan Reynolds Whyte, Sjaak van der Geest, and Anita Hardon (2002) argue that fruitful insights are gained by analyzing "the social life of medicines." Medicines have complicated biographies from their point of origin or production, transportation, prescription and purchase, and usages that endow them with complex social identities. Sams (2017, 1103, 1101) argues that health and healing are further complicated in Niger (and around the world) by the fact that medical choices are made to "mark affiliation to particular social groups and ideologies" and "perceptions of identity are used to analyse the efficacy of medication." Sams (2017, 1101) asserts that traditional healers and patients of Niger "interpret the efficacy of medication differently than biomedical professionals who prioritise a concern with the medication's fit with a disease rather than an individual." That is, for Nigériens medications can have social identities that are thought to be suitable only for people of specific social identities—even though those identities are fluid, flexible, contextual, and sometimes seemingly inconsistent. Furthermore, some Nigériens think that some illnesses are specific to ethnic groups and can be treated only with the medicine of those groups. I will analyze a quintessential example of a regional illness complex—heat–cold imbalance—that Nigériens think can best be treated with local traditional medicine in the following chapter. Indeed, Sams (2017, 1110) concluded, "diseases, as well as medication, were sometimes seen to have a social identity" among Hausa villagers of Kawari, Niger. In short, people, medications, and illnesses have social identities that must be balanced for effective healing in Niger.

There are some correlations between social identities and medical decision-making in Niamey. Nigériens with little or no secular education in French, especially those who grew up in rural areas, tend to trust and use traditional medicine more than medicine of other sectors. Nigériens for whom being Muslim is central to their identities tend to gravitate to Islamic medicine. Educated Nigériens, particularly those with wealth, are more likely than other Nigériens to trust biomedicine. However, I emphasize that there are many exceptions to this general pattern and the reality in Niamey is quite fluid. Most people in Niamey use all three medical sectors. Many uneducated people prefer biomedicine over other therapies. Many devout Muslims rarely use Islamic medicine. Many wealthy Francophone Nigériens use primarily traditional medicine. Women and men use traditional medicine and biomedicine roughly equally, but Islamic medicine in Niamey involves primarily men. I also found that Nigériens in Niamey of traditionally sedentary groups (Hausa, Zarma-Songhay, Mawri) are slightly more likely to trust biomedicine than Nigériens of traditionally nomadic groups (Tuareg, Fulani).

Finally, I emphasize the local and global mobility of patients, healers, medicines, and medical knowledge. Many Nigériens travel great distances at considerable cost—and sometimes risk as well—seeking therapeutic relief. Most traditional healers in Niamey walk the streets of the city with sacks or pushcarts advertising their services and selling their medicines (primarily plants). Many other itinerant traditional and Islamic healers travel circuits visiting a different village market day on each day of the week. Increasing numbers of Islamic healers of Niger travel to Saudi Arabia to study in Islamic universities, or with renowned healers, or for the hajj pilgrimage to Mecca, and return with new medical knowledge and medicines. Many Nigérien biomedical professionals are trained abroad, and some are foreigners. Much of the traditional medicine and Islamic medicine as well as all the biomedicine consumed in Niger is produced outside of Niger. Since patients, healers, and medicines circulate in Niger, so does healing knowledge. The dissemination of medical knowledge in Niamey is accelerating across all three therapeutic sectors through the increasing use of marketing technologies, including loudspeakers, billboards, CDs, radio, television, and social media. The mobilities of patients, healers, medicine, and medical knowledge are complexly intertwined. For example, Nigériens sometimes travel hundreds of kilometers or more to visit itinerant marabouts who treat them with medicines imported from Saudi Arabia. I argue that analyzing these forms of mobility as well as the interplay among them are key to understanding the complex nature of medical pluralism in Niger, or indeed any place in the world.

## CHAPTER 2

# Heat–Cold: The Quest for Balance in a Turbulent World

The most common health problems in Niamey involve an illness complex centered around the imbalance between "heat" and "cold." Focusing on this illness complex reveals critical insights on medical pluralism, medical mistrust, and underlying Nigérien cosmologies of health, illness, and healing. My extended discussion of heat–cold will: highlight its ubiquity in Niamey and the Sahel and speculate on what accounts for it, illustrate gender divisions and complementarity as well as ideas about sexuality, show that diffuse understandings of the etiologies and symptoms and overall complexity of heat–cold necessitate pluralistic therapeutic approaches, and argue that prevalence of heat–cold illnesses plays an important part in the endurance of the traditional medical sector. All of these factors, in combination with the mysterious, chronic nature of this illness complex and the general sense that it never be fully cured but only managed contributes to patients' mistrust of and "mistrustful dependency" (Pasquini 2023) on healers.

I draw from my own ethnographic research and from an excellent, nuanced—though small—body of scholarship to unpack the meanings of this central illness complex. Only two focused studies of heat–cold exist. The first is by Jean-Pierre Olivier de Sardan (1998) in his article "Illness Entities in West Africa." He focused on the complex among the Songhay-Zarma but emphasizes that variations of it are found across Niger (among Hausa, Fulani, Tuareg) and the West African Sahel (Mali, Burkina Faso, and the northern Sahel-Savanah regions of Benin, Côte d'Ivoire, Ghana, Nigeria, and Togo) among the Bambara, Mossi, Fulani, Soso, Dogon, and many others. Olivier de Sardan (1998, 213) emphasizes that "We have to remember that the *weyno*-and-*yeyni* ["hot"-and-"cold"] type is indeed very common, at least in

Sahelian West Africa, and it is a daily preoccupation for millions of people in towns or in villages. It has to be recognised for what it is—a central problem in public health, at least for ordinary people." The second extended analysis of heat–cold in the region—among Azawagh Arabs of northwestern Niger—is offered by Rebecca Popenoe (2004) in the chapter "Well-Being and Illness" of her book, *Feeding Desire*. Popenoe (2004, 172) emphasizes that it is difficult to make sense of this mysterious complex: "No one I asked could explain in fact what 'hot' and 'cold' meant in a way that clarified the logic of the system. The meanings of hot and cold were also unreflected upon because they are taken so much for granted by all ethnic groups in this part of the world, even if there are differences in how each group applies the system." In addition, L. Lewis Wall in *Hausa Medicine* (1988) offers some discussion of heat–cold among Hausa in Northern Nigeria, and other scholars of the region recognize its importance but do not focus on it (Rasmussen 2001, Sams 2019, Sams and Hyrinck 2021). Further afield, a similar complex was documented in Morocco by Greenwood (1992).

The question of why the heat–cold complex is so pervasive in the West Africa Sahel (even across pastoralists and agriculturalists, the most significant division in the region) is open to interpretation in part because its origins are also open to interpretation. One plausible explanation is that the heat–cold complex was an element of the Islamic medicine that began arriving in the region 1,000 years ago. Recall the expansive definition of "Islamic medicine" that I used earlier as including medical principles absorbed from various cultures wherever Muslim communities have resided over time, including principles and practices that are not included in the Qur'an or Hadiths. Evidence suggests that Muslim communities adopted the heat–cold complex from the Greek humoral system during medieval times (Abdallah 1992, 177; Campbell 2013; Popenoe 2004, 172), and that later Arab Muslims brought it with them to West Africa. Popenoe (2004, 172) argues that over time in West Africa (and other places where the system traveled), "The original Greek four-category system of hot, cold, wet, and dry has been reworked and simplified . . . to focus on heat and coldness," though there is still evidence of the importance of "wet" and "dry" in Niamey and elsewhere in the region. A second plausible explanation is that the heat–cold complex existed in West Africa before the arrival of Islam. Third, both of those explanations are plausible; that is, West Africans may have recognized and assimilated the heat–cold principles of "Islamic medicine" because they were similar to their own preexisting ideas. Indeed, the histories of traditional and Islamic medicine have been intertwined for so long in Niger that in some cases it makes no sense to differ-entiate them and more sense to refer to "traditional Islamic medicine," which is another important dimension of medical pluralism in Niger.

Health, for Nigériens, is all about balancing or harmonizing relationships between otherwise opposing forces and people—most importantly, "heat" and "cold," and men and women. Imbalance leads to illnesses, involving both diverse internal symptoms and external visible symptoms with consequences that range from minor annoyances to death. Popenoe (2004,171) makes sev-eral crucial points to open her discussion of "heat" and "cold": "Despite the terminology, the categories have little to do with temperature, but rather represent two overarching categories that each encompass many different qualities, not least those to do with sexual desire and desirability . . . balance between hot and cold is a condition not just of personal health but of the gen-eral well-being of the world." While there is a great deal of overlap across eth-nic groups of the region in conceptualizations of "heat" and "cold," there are also important differences between them. The multiethnic and transethnic urban setting of Niamey in my research contributed to my confusion about "heat" and "cold." It is difficult enough to comprehend the complex within one ethnic group because no two people see it exactly the same way. The heat–cold complex is structured by gender, though not exactly in the same ways across ethnic groups in the Sahel. "Heat" and "cold" are experienced by men and women in overlapping as well as very different ways. Regarding the latter, only women experience the "heat" of pregnancy, of energy surging inside the body in the creation of a new life. Furthermore, food classification systems vary by ethnicity. For example, Hausa (Wall 1988, 297) think of tomatoes as "cold" and use them to treat "heat," whereas Azawagh Arabs (Popenoe 2004, 173) regard tomatoes as "hot" because they are associated with a foreign world outside of the Sahara.

Popenoe's nuanced, thick description of "heat" and "cold" is focused on Azawagh Arabs, but my research indicates her conclusions are generally valid in Niamey and the wider region. She explains that "Heat is generally a quality of heat enclosed in the body, and cold a quality of the body being too open . . . heat is also a quality of energy concentrated, whereas cold is a quality of energy dissipated" (Popenoe, 172, 173). Because women are open and men are closed, women are generally thought of as "cold" and men as "hot." However, this is not a simply binary. Azawagh Arab women want "to be a little hot, for example, to be sexy" (Popenoe 2004, 173). They can, however, become "too hot" for vari-ous reasons, especially pregnancy, after which they are uniquely vulnerable to being "too cold." Azawagh Arab men tend to be "hot," and while their semen is considered "cold," sex and sexuality are "heat"-oriented. As I found in my interviews and conversations and as is highlighted in the literature, too much cold in Amazagh is associated with sexually transmitted diseases and genital discharges in women and men. Sexually transmitted diseases are particularly dreaded in the Sahel, because ultimately women's greatest health fear is infertility (Cooper 2019; Moussa 2023). This is generally true of men, too.

Wall (1988, 147) documented that among Hausa, "In symbolic terms women are classified as cold (*sanyi*), while men are hot (*zahi*)." However, both women and men can suffer from "cold" and both women and men can suffer from "heat." Each gender can weaken the other, especially through sexual relations. Women can make men too cold, and men can make women too hot. Women's efforts to protect themselves from men's heat can overdo it and make them too cold. Men's efforts to protect themselves from women's cold can overdo it and make them too hot.

The primary healer-vendors of medicine for "heat" on the streets of Niamey are women (of a range of ethnicities of Niger, Benin, and Togo) on foot who carry repurposed water bottles with a liquid mixture of herbs that can be dispensed on the spot in small plastic cups. This is the only medicine that they sell, unlike most street healers, and they sell it to both men and women on the streets of Niamey. Most market transactions are perfunctory, with a standard rate of 200 CFA for basic "heat medicine." Other more complicated cases of "heat" involve more specialized treatments that can cost 1,000 CFA or much more, depending on negotiations between healers and clients. Some patients trust a regular healer to treat "heat," but most rely on steady stream of women healers who follow regular footpaths and pass by where they work or hang out daily. Other men and women healers sell the raw botanical ingredients to clients who prefer to make their own mixes for "heat" and "cold" at home. Azawagh Arabs follow a similar pattern: "When both men and women fall ill, they turn first to this female-dominated form of therapy [for heat–cold], and only if several attempts at treatment have failed does an ill person turn to the more expensive, male-controlled Islamic therapies" (Popenoe 2004, 185).

Women's role as the primary everyday vendors of medicine for "heat" reveals gendered inequality as well as tensions and complementarity and women's power. On the one hand, women are relegated to specializing in an illness complex for which, as mentioned earlier, "There is no real cure . . . the feeling that this disease can never be definitively cured is widely shared" (Olivier de Sardan, 1998, 194, 195). Similarly, Popenoe (2004, 175) explains

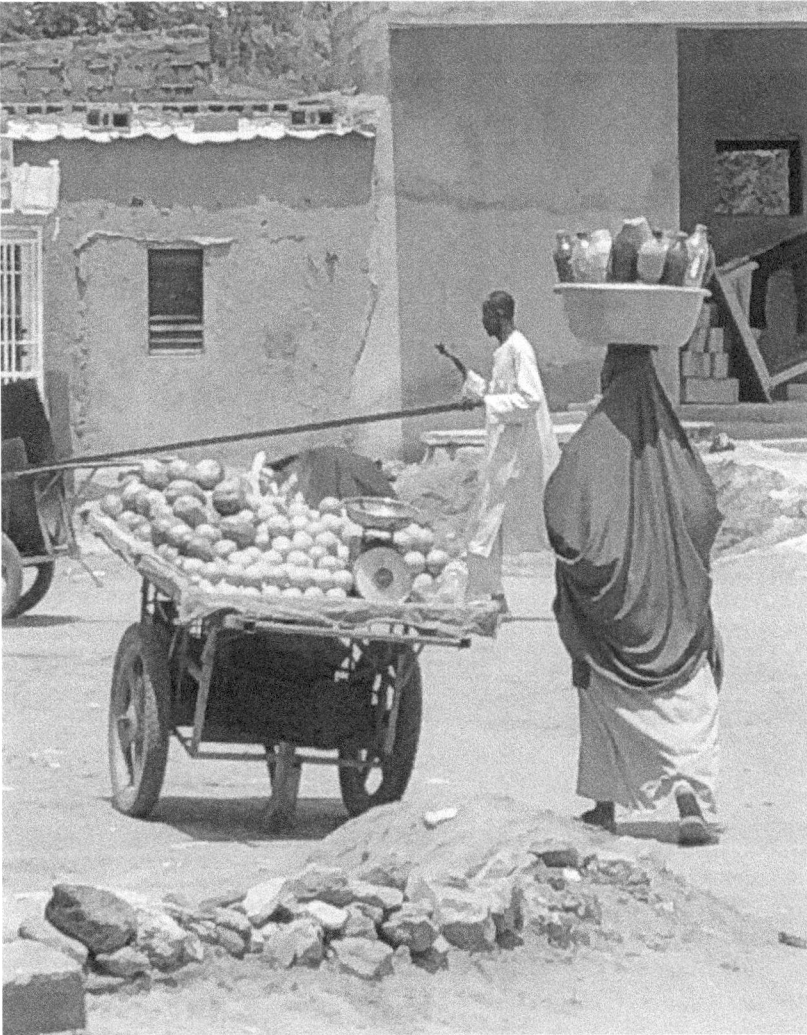

Figure 2.1. Healer with heat–cold imbalance medicines. Photo by author.

that "There are numerous ways to seek and achieve balance, but also endless opportunities for the balance to be thrown off." On the other hand, men trust women as the "go-to" source for medicine for "heat." As one middle-aged Hausa man put it, echoing the opinions of several others, "Women make us sick with 'heat' because of all the hot spices and oil they use in their cooking

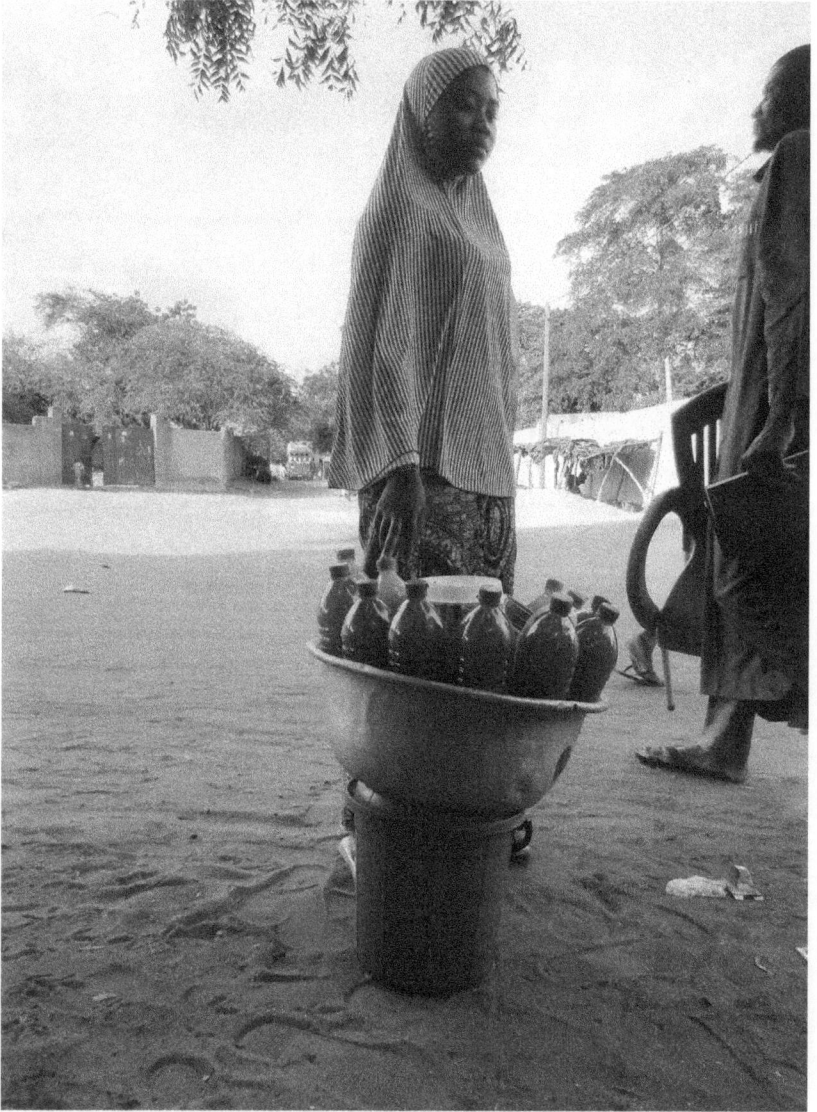

Figure 2.2. Heat–cold imbalance medicines. Photo by author.

and then they profit from our suffering by selling us medicine that makes us feel better, but only temporarily." The thought that healers would go out of business if they actually cured everyone is a widespread source of medical mistrust in Niger and globally. His Zarma friend replied, "Women are devious, we cannot live with them, but we cannot live without them." Many other men simply explained that women are most suited to treating "heat" since women are associated with cold. Because women are particularly vulnerable to being too hot (especially during pregnancy) as well being too cold (especially while menstruating, during sexual relations, postpartum), they typically pay more attention to maintaining heat–cold balance than men do. Women's power—subtle but undeniable, though steadily eroding in increasingly patriarchal Niger due to the recent rise of Salafi forms of Islam in Niger—rests in their knowledge of heat–cold and the trust that men and women place in women healers to handle most treatments for the most common, and, when we include its myriad manifestations, most important illness in Niamey.

Women and men enjoy heat–cold medical transactions more than any other medical transactions on the street. (Actually, there is little or no joy or pleasure in any of the other medical interactions in Niamey.) Women take pride in their occupation that allows them to independently earn modest but steady and family-supporting incomes in public spaces—which is very unusual in highly gender-segregated Niger. Nigérien Muslim men enjoy briefly chatting and politely flirting with these women in these transactions, especially the Christian and animist Beninoise and Togolaise women who tend to be far less reserved than Muslim Nigérien women. Women reciprocate, but for them it may simply be a nuisance that they have to endure as part of the cost of being in business.[1] These interactions are somewhat exceptional because women do not typically interact much with men outside of their families on the streets of Niamey. Women often require the assistance of male customers to help them lower their heavy tin basins full of bottled medicines and later to help them lift them back atop their heads—providing unusual opportunities for women and men to come into close, physical contact. While I observed the pleasure that men and women take in these interactions, reading Popenoe's analysis allowed me to understand the deeper reasons behind it. Even though she focused on Azawagh Arabs in rural Niger who make up about only one percent of Nigériens, her insights make sense for interpreting the interactions that I observed on the streets of Niamey, primarily among Hausa and

Zarma-Songhay. She explains that "The public discourse about hot and cold is one of food, illnesses, plants, and cooking methods, but . . . the underlying text is one of sexuality" (Popenoe 2004, 182).

Women sell "cold" medicine for women primarily in the private compounds of Niamey, though sometimes in public spaces as well. This makes sense because women trust women healers far more than male healers, and because even though "cold" can catch men, "cold" is first and foremost a women's illness since its primary cause is childbirth. Nevertheless, medical gender mixing is common as women healers sell heat and cold medicine to women and men; and men sell heat and cold medicine to women and men.

Nigériens describe the *causes* and *symptoms* of and *treatments* for "heat" and "cold" in a wide kaleidoscopic variety of ways. *Causes*: In Niger, "heat" and "cold" are interpreted as naturalistic illnesses by Songhay-Zarma (Olivier de Sardan 1998, 204), Tuareg (Rasmussen 2001, 42), and Hausa (Sams and Hyrinck 2020, 31; Wall 1988, 187). In contrast, among Azawagh Arabs of Niger spirits (as well as naturalistic causes) are associated with "heat" (Popenoe 2004, 172). "Heat" and "cold" illnesses are caused by imbalances or having too much "heat" or too much "cold." My interviewees—across a wide range of ethnicities—indicate that heat is caused primarily by eating too many spicy foods and sitting too long especially on hard wooden benches, whereas cold is caused by consumption of cold liquids and exposure to cold temperatures, especially the damp cold of the rainy season. Babies and postpartum mothers are thought to be particularly vulnerable to threat of being too cold, and thus babies are typically dressed in sweaters and knit hats even on 105-degree days, and among the Hausa and others new mothers take extremely hot baths twice a day for 40 days (Cooper 2019, 163; Smith 1954, 126; Wall 1988, 230).

Olivier de Sardan (1998) observes that among Songhay-Zarma, heat (*weyno*) is seen as "chronic, progressive, and hereditary," and has many causes and manifestations, citing an expert healer who recognizes and treats 12 different forms (1998, 201). These include sexual transmission from women to men (Olivier de Sardan 1998, 204), the irregular eating of meals, and relatively recent dietary changes such as "the current over-use of sugar (formerly a rare commodity), groundnut oil (introduced in huge quantities under colonisation and refined locally) and salt (sea salt replacing local salts, and the widespread use of Maggi spice [a Nestlé product high in sodium, including monosodium glutamate])" (Olivier de Sardan (1998, 205). Sitting is also considered a leading source of *weyno* among Songhay-Zarma, especially for those who sit for long periods of time on wooden benches but also for taxi drivers with relatively soft seats (Olivier de Sardan, 1998, 207) as my interviews across ethnic groups also indicated. Sams and Hrynick (2020, 31) report that the causes of heat include "over-exposure to sun, too much sugar or tobacco or oil in meals, not eating well or eating at irregular times," whereas "cold"—"which is sometimes seen as a more advanced version of *zahi*"—is "caused by giving birth, can be transmitted by women to men, or arise in men who do not fully ejaculate." Rasmussen (2001, 42) found that Tuareg believe that hot illnesses are caused by eating too much sugar or "bad food" such as potatoes, a cultural particularity.

*Symptoms*: I found that "heat" is far more commonly treated than "cold" in Niamey, but this may be due to my focus on street healers and patients and the gendered nature of the heat–cold complex. Hemorrhoids are by far the most often reported symptom of "heat" in my urban multi-ethnic research, but my interviewees describe a diverse set of symptoms including a wide range of gastrointestinal pain and problems, blood in the stool, general weakness including sexual impotence, and loss of appetite. Other symptoms of "heat" include "fever, chills, eye problems, impotence, stomach problems, diarrhea, articulation pain, regular headaches, mental instability"; whereas "cold" can cause "urinary problems, genital discharge, fever, pain in lower limbs and stomach, shrinking of male sex," according to Sams and Hrynick (2020, 31). For the Songhay-Zarma, there are many types of "heat," but most are centered in the pelvic region from the navel to the lower back and involve internal and external symptoms including hemorrhoids, blood in the stool or urine, constipation, diarrhea, vomiting, and jaundice (Olivier de Sardan 1998, 195, 205). Cold (*yeyni*) among the Songhay-Zarma includes three forms involving persistent pain in the bones, flesh, and belly (Olivier de Sardan 1998, 195).

Wall (1988, 190) argues that for Hausa "The effects of heat (*zafi*) are felt mainly on the external body and are generally not as important in pathological explanations as are the effects of cold (*sanyi*)," and reports different sets of symptoms. According to Wall's (1988, 190) research, "heat" typically manifests itself as sharp pain on the external body, such as hemorrhoids (*basur*) or "painful rashes and eruptions on the skin, such as smallpox (*agana*), chicken pox (*karambau, 'kanda*), or measles (*ba'kon dauro, 'kyanda*)" or leprosy (*kutruta*). Among Tuareg, "heat" is felt in the middle of the stomach, whereas "cold" is felt in the bladder (Rasmussen 2001, 74). Wall (1988, 297) found that "cold" is particularly insidious—echoing Sams and Hrynick's conclusion that "cold" is "a more advanced version of *zahi*"—as it increases "phlegm inside the body, producing head and chest colds, killing the blood, sapping a man's strength, and causing a variety of internal ailments." Wall (1988, 189) notes that "*amo-sani* is the Hausa term referring to the most long-lasting and disruptive effects of *sanyi*." *Amosani* is complex: it can occur in the joints (leading to arthritis), in the head (leading to headaches, loss of teeth, deafness, and blindness), or in the abdomen (leading to a variety of gastrointestinal ailments). Cold can move from one part of the body to another (Wall 1988, 189) and although it "affects the internal organs, it may lead to external swellings as it works its way outward" (Wall 1988, 297). Furthermore, a person's body can be "hot" in one place and simultaneously "cold" in another (Popenoe 2004, 181). The heat–cold complex is not a simple binary. "Heat" can also lead to the buildup of "dead blood" just as "cold" can. Both "heat" and "cold" can also involve external symptoms, such as rashes, acne, and shingles.

*Treatments*: Nigériens seek treatments for heat–cold illnesses from all three medical sectors, traditional, Islamic, and biomedical. This illness complex illustrates that part of navigating these sectors involves accumulating knowledge about which is best suited to treating certain ailments. Nigériens prefer traditional medicine over medicine from other sectors for the treatment of heat–cold illnesses in most cases. Many Nigériens think that they can prophylactically avoid "heat" and "cold" by eating healthy food, in reasonable portions, at very regular times (Olivier de Sardan 1998, 205). In addition, many of the people I interviewed indicated that one should not get too "high" or too "low" in terms of behavior, demeanor, and emotions. They explained that impatience, loud arguments, and anger can lead to physical "heat" illnesses. Popenoe (2004, 180) documented that among Azawagh Arabs, "Outside the time of pregnancy, the negotiation of heat and cold in the body is still a pervasive everyday concern, and one that requires constant adjustment of foods." They are particularly attuned to very subtle differences in food preparation that change the "hotness" or "coldness" of foods. For example, Popenoe (2004, 181) explains that among Azawagh Arabs millet porridge is generally considered a "colder" food, but there are many varieties of it "on a continuum of hot to cold, based on how finely the millet is pounded, how it is cooked (boiled, steamed, in the ground, not cooked), and whether or not it is sifted."

A diverse range of medicines for "heat" include "drinks made with the powder of local plants, biomedical treatments such as Flagyl (metronida-zole)[2], and lion urine, purchased from the National Museum, may be used as a treatment in advanced cases" (Sams and Hrynich (2020, 31). I found that tonics are by far the most commonly used treatments for "heat" and "cold." Typically, they are purgatives. My research indicates these include a wide range of plant ingredients that are dissolved in water, such as the leaves of *kenkeliba, gao,* and *gaiza* trees; the leaves and flowers of *sabara, kargo, derga,* and *gujiya kasa* shrubs; and the roots of *goda* bushes. I am not a botanist, but I know that there are many other plants that are used to treat "heat" and "cold." Furthermore, all the people that I interviewed—mobile women street vendors, traditional herbalists, and people who make their own concoctions at home—indicate that they use materials from two to four or more different kinds of plants. This means that there are hundreds—probably thousands—of different versions of medicine for "heat" and "cold" in Niamey. Wall (1988, 297) observes that among Hausa, heat is treated—internally and externally—with cool foods like honey and tomatoes, whereas cold is treated with hot foods such as a variety of spicy peppers.

Among Songhay-Zarma there are various remedies for "cold" including "tying the affected limb above and below the painful area; singeing with a red-hot iron (*kagatu*); cupping [and bloodletting] with a horn (*hilli*); immersion in river water up to the neck for certain period" (Olivier de Sardan 1998, 195-6). Treatments for "cold" also include "plants, Koranic verses, amulets, and bush animals (skins or meat)" (Sams and Hrynick (2020, 31). Rasmussen (200, 56) similarly reports that among Tuareg to restore balance and health hot illnesses require cold food such as millet, whereas cold illnesses require hot food such as dates, drawing from indigenous cultural logics of what makes certain things "hot" others "cold." Cupping and bloodletting are used to remove "dead blood" caused by either "heat" or "cold" (as well as other problems) across ethnic groups. On Facebook, Sheikh Ahmad Ibn Hamza, an Islamic healer of Kaduna (Northern Nigeria) posted an advertisement on January 5, 2025, in the group "j'acheté [sic], vend, et troc en Niamey," claiming to have medicine to treat 60 symptoms of "cold."

I suspect that readers are confused about "heat" and "cold." I am too! Sams (2017, 1106) refers to "heat" as a "local disease with no biomedical equivalent." "Heat" and "cold" defy translation into biomedical terminology and understanding; "From a biomedical point of view, they seem to be an amalgamation of very diverse and often complex pathologies" (Olivier de Sardan 1998, 194). Popenoe (2004, 175–176) argues that the logics behind heat-cold thinking are radically different from those in biomedicine. Many Nigériens are also confused by "heat" and "cold" and they clearly hold a wide range of thoughts about their causes, symptoms, and treatments. This complexity simultaneously leads to mistrust of healers and reliance on them since the illness complex is difficult to understand on one's own. As such, it is a prime example of what Pasquini (2023) identified as a relationship of "mis-trustful dependency" between patients and healers. Indeed, as Olivier de Sar-dan (1998, 200) explains for the Songhay-Zarma—and this is generally true for Nigériens—there is no "unifying theory whatsoever concerning the vari-ous forms of ["heat"] *weyno*, or any principle governing the whole entity . . ." These words echo those of Popenoe cited at the opening of this discussion and my own challenging experience in seeking to understand heat–cold.

The overall complexity and mysterious nature of the heat–cold complex, including the fact that it can move in the body and symptoms progress over time and thus require different treatments, virtually necessitates pluralistic medical approaches. Traditional therapies are preferred overall, but biomedical drugs are also widely used to treat various symptoms, while Islamic medicine is only occasionally used. Given that heat–cold may have arrived in the West African Sahel with the arrival of Muslim traders and scholars, as I suggested earlier, the fact that Nigériens use primarily traditional medicines to treat may represent an important cultural shift, or the indigenization of "Islamic medi-cine" in the region. Furthermore, many of the symptoms of "heat" and "cold," which are natural illnesses for Nigérien ethnic groups except for Azawagh Arabs, are the same symptoms of illnesses that are caused supernaturally (by spirits, sorcerers, and witches) and socio-emotionally (by envy, rivalry, and other conflict). This means therapies from across healing modalities are used. Popenoe's (2004, 174) explanation of the navigation of therapeutic pluralism among Azawagh Arabs parallels what I found in Niamey: "Many diseases can come from a surplus of either hot or cold, and only by symptoms' reaction to a known hot or cold medicine can one know the nature of a disease, hot treating cold, and cold, hot." This process can also lead to the conclusion that an illness is neither "heat" nor "cold" related, which in turn can lead a healer to look for other causes, or in some cases to refer patients to biomedical specialists. Sim-ilarly, as described earlier, physicians sometimes refer patients to traditional healers, including those who specialize in the treatment of heat–cold. Medical pluralism in Niamey is multidirectional.

Most Nigériens in Niamey across classes, levels of educational attainment, genders, and ethnicities think that "heat" and "cold" responds best to tradi-tional medicine. Olivier de Sardan (1998, 206–207) argues that "The use of modern health services, the ready availability of pharmaceutical drugs, edu-cation in schools—these different factors, largely synonymous with urban life, have hardly had any effect on the importance of ["heat"] in popular diagnosis and medication . . . and is quite striking." He observed this more than 25 years ago, and my research showed that it still largely holds true.

The prevalence of heat–cold illnesses in part accounts for the endurance of the traditional medical sector in Niamey and in the Sahel. It is not only people that have social identities, illnesses and medications also have social identities and all must be balanced for effective healing. Perhaps more than other illness, heat–cold imbalance is seen by most Nigériens as a Nigérien complex requiring traditional local medicines to alleviate. Many times, over the years, I was warned by Nigérien friends to never take *maganin zahi* (heat medicine). They told me that it would not kill me, but it would not help me either, and that I would likely suffer severe stomach pain because it does not "fit" a white American. (Sams [2017, 1101] was similarly warned against buying the cheap versions of malaria drugs used by most local Nigériens on the grounds that they would not "fit" or work for her son and was advised to purchase a premium Western version.) Nevertheless, because virtually all Nigériens I know take *maganin zahi* occasionally or regularly (once a week or more) and extol its virtues, and due to the curiosity of a participant observer suffering from bloating and constipation—quintessential symptoms of *zahi*—I tried it once. I was glad that I did it from the comfort of my home, as I had several rounds of urgent diarrhea. By the next morning I was no longer bloated and constipated but wiped out and wondered if I would have been better off if I had taken pharmaceuticals or just rested.

In 2023, two longtime friends independently and unbeknown to each other told me virtually identical stories about their therapeutic trajectories during their experiences with "heat." Though seemingly anecdotal, they illustrate widespread opinions across social classes expressed in free-flowing conversations and intensive interviews with a wide range of people. Both are middle-aged professional men with master's degrees—one is married to a biomedical physician and the other to a biomedical pharmacist. The men regularly trust biomedicine for a variety of illnesses, but they also regularly use traditional and Islamic medicines. Each described his primary problem as severe hemorrhoids and sought treatment in hospitals, where they were prescribed various pharmaceuticals and surgery was strongly recommended. They tried the drugs and reported they felt no relief and declined the surgical option.

Next, they sought out well-known traditional herbalists, a man in a nearby village and a woman in Ouagadougou, Burkina Faso. These are expert specialists in the treatment of "heat" with knowledge and capabilities above and beyond the typical women vendors on the street and generalist herbalist men and women vendors who sell "heat medicine" among dozens of other remedies for other illnesses. Each reported returning to health in a week, expressed their relief about having forgone surgery (and its costs, recovery time, and possible complications), and emphasized that in the future they will only trust traditional medicine to treat "heat." This is a good example of the contextual mistrust of biomedicine. These men trust biomedicine about as much overall as traditional and Islamic medicine, but not for "heat." While both men found relief at least temporarily, drawing from the overall evidence presented in this discussion, I argue that the social context in which Nigériens typically regard "heat" and "cold" as mysterious, chronic (and in some cases hereditary) conditions for which there are no permanent remedies contributes to a social climate of pervasive skepticism, doubt, and mistrust about not only heat–cold but also about healing in general in Niger. Ambiguities about the most common ailment and therapies for it are connected to pervasive medical mistrust in Niamey in general.

Following Olivier de Sardan (1998, 206–207), I have emphasized continuity in understandings of and therapies for the heat–cold complex. However, core ideas may be shifting, namely ideas about the dangers of coldness. When I first lived in Niger in the 1980s and 1990s, virtually no Nigériens drank cold water. People explained to me that they regarded ice water as dangerous to health, not only because of the immediate sharp dental pain that would result—many Nigériens suffer with chronic dental pain—but more importantly that it could lead to serious "cold" illness. Beginning in the 2000s, after the practice diffused from Nigeria, Nigérien street vendors began selling "sachet water," 500-milliliter clear plastic bags of ice-cold water (Keough and Youngstedt 2019). It was cleverly marketed as modern, clean, and pure. Indeed, it is most commonly referred to as pure water or *piya wata*—a "Hausafication" of Nigerian English. It took about a decade, but by the mid-2010s the popularity of sachet water exploded, and now it is the most common source of drinking water for people who are away from home. Middle-aged and older Nigériens typically still refuse cold water—though they sometimes buy sachet water and just wait for it to warm up—but I also know many in their 50s and 60s who began drinking cold sachet water regularly just a few years ago after never having drunk it before. Younger Nigériens have collective amnesia regarding cultural avoidance of cold water. They love it. I do not know if this is leading to changing thoughts about the dangers of "cold" in a broader sense, but I suspect that it will. As Falen (2018, 18, original emphasis) argues, "African ritual and thought *do* allow for self-reflection, critique, and even the abandonment of theory. Within African systems of thought lies the potential for dramatic change and transformation." In the coming years, this may lead to changing ideas about "cold" in Niamey or decreasing attributions of illness to overdrinking cold water.

I have struggled for many years to make sense of the nature of and treatments for "heat" and "cold" in Niger. For a long time, it seemed simple to me and not worthy of much attention. It made sense to me that eating "too much" spicy food could lead to "hot" digestive problems and hemorrhoids, smoking "too many" cigarettes lead to "hot" respiratory ailments, and a postpartum mother would feel "cold." I finally have a better sense of why Nigériens avoid getting caught in the rain if all possible even during (what for me are) very hot days temperature-wise when it feels refreshing to stand in the rain. "Wet" is linked with "cold," especially the damp cold of the rainy season. Still, I think I am only beginning to understand heat–cold, and I wonder if there is more that I do not understand than what I do understand about it. I hope that readers have a better understanding of the heat–cold complex now than when they began reading this, and can clearly appreciate that this complex is part of the taken-for-grant reality of Nigériens, that it clearly is about gender and sexuality explicitly and implicitly, and that its prevalence and complicated nature contribute to medical mistrust and medical pluralism, and especially to the enduring relevance of the traditional medical sector in Niger.

Popenoe (2004, 175, 184) offers an expansive interpretation of "heat" and "cold," a proverbial Rosetta stone for unlocking their deeper meaning, that warrants a lengthy citation.

> The qualities of hot and cold inhere not only in diseases and in [traditional, Islamic, and modern] medicines, but in all plants, all bodily conditions, sexuality, the weather, and even, to some extent, history. The forces of hot and cold are ubiquitous . . . Unifying the human body, the environment, the spirit world, and social life in a cohesive universe, the qualities of hot and cold entail all of God's creations are mutually dependent and interacting . . . The dualism of hot and cold by which Allah has ordered his creations, be they plant, animal, or mineral, necessarily serves as the preeminent dualism by which he ordered humanity, male and female. Hot and cold are nature's expression of the sexuality that pulls male and female together to satisfy the

most base human passions as well as the most noble human aims, to
be fruitful and multiply in one's own and in Allah's name.

Recall that Popenoe's research focused on Azawagh Arabs in rural northwestern Niger. My research in Niamey—primarily among Hausa, Zarma-
Songhay, Mawri, Tuareg, and Fulani—suggests Popenoe's insightful synthesis
is generally valid among Nigériens. Popenoe's synthesis meshes neatly with
the holistic sense among Nigériens that physical, spiritual, socio-emotional
health are intertwined. However, I never encountered anyone in my research
who summarized the deep meaning of heat–cold in the way that Popenoe
does. None of the Nigériens I encountered in Niamey spoke about heat–cold
in a broad, abstract way. Very few people that I talked with explicitly linked
heat–cold with sexuality. Nevertheless, it was there all along implicitly, in the
subtle pleasure that men take in buying heat medicine from women. One of
the hallmarks of the discipline of anthropology is the perspective that sometimes "outsiders"—expert anthropologists who engage in long-term research
and understand the nuances of local languages such as Popenoe—can "see
the forest through the trees" more clearly than "insiders" can, especially in
situations involving what are everyday, taken-for-granted realties for locals
such as heat–cold.

# CHAPTER 3

---

## Developing and Perpetuating Mistrust

"That shit will kill you, because all *bokaye* are liars."
"How can this company be selling five-liter containers of Zam Zam
    water [holy water]?"
"Corona tests and vaccinations were designed to sterilize African
    Muslims."

I heard these comments regarding medical mistrust and similar ones on a
regular basis, in interviews and in casual conversation in the past few years
in Niamey. The first comment refers to specific types of traditional plant
medicines and a particular type of healers, *bokaye*, who are herbalists who
also sometimes work with spirits in therapy. Although the words are extreme,
the speaker in fact relies on many types of traditional medicine. Furthermore,
I would not be surprised if he sometimes consults with *bokaye* but is reluctant to share this to protect his public reputation as a good Muslim as locally
defined. He thus illustrates the common practice of men and women in Niger
critiquing forms of medicine that they actually use.

Nigérien Muslims and Muslims everywhere regard the Zam Zam well of
Mecca as the source of the most potent, holy, healing water in the world.
The man who posed the second question trusts holy water and Islamic medicine in general. However, he and many Nigériens express concern about its
commodification and are aware that pilgrims are permitted to bring home
one five-liter container of Zam Zam water. Thus, his mistrust was focused on
the purveyor who was advertising Zam Zam for sale in an online Facebook
group. A friend of the man who asked this question posed a follow-up: "If it
is authentic Zam Zam water then why would someone sell it instead of just

drinking it?" He is mistrustful of both the authenticity of the holy water and the integrity of the vendor.

The woman who made the third comment was sharing one of several widely circulating rumors in Niamey regarding COVID-19. Nigérien perspectives on COVID-19 reveal a deep-rooted fear and mistrust of public health crisis campaigns and of global "racial capitalism" (Robinson 1983). She, like many Nigériens, mistrusts the WHO and the Nigérien state, especially their emergency health policies that are seen as unnecessary and disruptive, although she does trust biomedical pharmaceuticals and most standard vaccinations for the healthcare of her children. As is common in Niger, she reconciles seemingly opposed positions.

These three short comments—with some contextualization—illustrate *seven* of the core themes of this chapter. I closely examine medical mistrust among patients in Niamey, considering mistrust of healers, medicines, and health institutions and principles across traditional, Islamic, and biomedical sectors.

*First, medical mistrust is pervasive and permeates the healing cultures of Niamey.* People in Niamey express mistrust of each medical sector in different though often overlapping ways with striking frequency. Medical skepticism, doubt, and mistrust are regular topics of everyday conversation in the city.

*Second, medical mistrust and trust among Nigériens exist on a continuum.* Medical mistrust and trust can be absolute extremes among Nigériens. Most Nigériens thoroughly mistrust COVID-19 vaccines, for reasons that I will explain in Chapter 6. However, while medical trust can be absolute, it rarely is for Nigériens. Instead, it is possible to identify degrees of trust, or to think of continuum between full trust and full mistrust. The man who said "That shit will kill you" does not reject all traditional medicine, nor does the woman who expressed fear of COVID-19 tests and vaccinations reject biomedicine as a whole. Furthermore, among Nigériens, one might not trust any healers but might not have any choice but to take a risk, such as trying to find the healer who one mistrusts the least.

*Third, mistrust is multifaceted and contextual, involving social relations and calculations of advantage.* Mistrust is also an attitude and perspective for negotiating indeterminacy. We must ask exactly who or what is mistrusted in context. Sometimes Nigériens mistrust people, either as individuals, such as a specific traditional healer (*boka*, singular) and a particular vendor of Zam Zam water, or as a type or group, such as the man who said "all *bokaye* are liars." All three speakers expressed mistrust of specific medicines or specific tests and vaccinations. The woman who commented on COVID-19 mistrusts the principles and practices of global health institutions and the state.

*Fourth, Nigériens mistrust the commodification of health care and medicine*, as illustrated by the doubts about selling Zam Zam water. This mistrust of monetization crosscuts traditional, Islamic, and biomedical sectors. Nigériens have always paid healers, in kind or in cash. They do not expect therapy to be free, though they sometimes do not mind when it occasionally is free, as it has been since 2006 for children under the age of five years and for prenatal and laboring women (Heller 2019, 134).[1] In contrast, Nigériens sometimes mistrust medical services provided free of charge, such as polio vaccinations (Sams and Hrynick 2020, 20), precisely because they are offered free of charge, suspecting that there must be a "catch." Nigériens fear that healers are increasingly motivated by earning money, which in turn has made them less committed to healing people.

*Fifth, Nigériens are rarely paralyzed by medical mistrust.* Medical mistrust constitutes a form of engagement with the therapeutic landscape in Niamey. Each of the people quoted make use of medicines from medical sectors that they also vehemently criticize in particular ways. Nigériens regularly use medicines and other therapies that they do not fully trust. In this chapter, I will argue that power, risk, mistrust, and trust regarding health care are not static but instead are negotiated and renegotiated, in continuously shifting contexts.

*Sixth, Nigériens widely think that healers can—and sometimes do—use their knowledge to accidently or purposely harm or kill people.* The first and third comments reveal this fear, which is an extreme form of medical mistrust.

*Seventh, to varying extents representatives and healers of each medical sector seek to discredit healers and medicines of other sectors.* This behavior fuels medical mistrust in Niamey as this rhetoric is widely shared among residents of the city. It illustrates that medical pluralism contributes to medical mistrust in Niamey.

## What Are Mistrust and Trust in Medical Matters and Why Does It Matter?

Medical mistrust and trust are conjoined. Neither exists without the other, and yet they are not the same. Jaiswal and Halkitis (2019, 80) argue that "Mistrust is not merely the opposite of trust but is more than simply the absence of trust; mistrust often refers to the belief that the entity that is the object of mistrust is acting against one's best interest or well-being." In contrast, Boyas and Valera (2011, 144) offer a definition of medical trust that I find useful as involving "faith that the health care provider will act in accordance with the patient's best interest, derived from the physician's medical values of fidelity, honesty, beneficence, and competence." Nigériens hope that traditional, Islamic, and biomedical healers share these core ethics. A vast body of literature in medical anthropology and health sciences emphasizes the importance of trust in health care, focuses on how health care providers can earn trust, and documents negative consequences of medical mistrust. Indeed, some minimal level of trust is required for a patient to try a healer's medicine, though trust always involves risking disappointment. Pasquini (2023, 580) argues that this literature often overlooks the fundamental reality that the healer–patient relationship is an inherently asymmetrical power relationship, involving disparity of knowledge and power, and therefore that we must consider "mistrust, not as an absence or a destructive force, but as an intrinsic aspect of power relationships in healthcare, a 'mistrustful dependency' in which risk management tools are used to navigate asymmetric care relationships."

Mühlfried's (2018, 11) central theoretical point about the dialectical tension between mistrust and trust is a useful perspective for understanding the medical ethos of Niamey: "Both trust and mistrust are attitudes of engagement . . . which is why they cannot be understood as opposites . . . They both emerge in situations of uncertainty. Trust also does not necessarily disappear with advent of mistrust." He continues by explaining that "On a more abstract level, trust and mistrust have to be seen as mutually constitutive: mistrust needs to be possible for trust to come into existence" (Mühlfried 2018, 11). Hence, as I have already mentioned, I argue that medical mistrust and trust among Nigériens exists on a continuum. Mistrust and trust involve cognitive and emotional dimensions and mutual interactions. This chapter investigates the roots of medical mistrust (and trust) in Niger. It sets the context for Chapter 4, which examines the ways that Nigériens navigate the therapeutic landscape in Niamey despite pervasive medical mistrust, and for Chapter 5, which focuses on the strategies used by healers across medical sectors to earn the trust of patients. Medical mistrust and trust matter because these are key variables in medical decision-making in Niger and universally. Trusting the wrong healer or medicine can have lethal consequences. By the same token, medical mistrust—such as declining a vaccine—can lead to premature death for oneself and others.

I argue that medical mistrust is a useful perspective when medical knowledge is contested and medical outcomes and the future in general are highly uncertain—as they are in Niger and many other places today. Akin to my approach to the history of medical pluralism in Niger in Chapter 1, I will tack back and forth between the present and the past, and then show how the historical origins of medical mistrust influence contemporary mistrust. I begin with an overview of intersecting precarities today in Niger and argue that intense ambiguity about so many important things in life—health, jobs, safety, rain, stability—contributes to medical doubt, skepticism, and mistrust. Then I will turn to a discussion of the dialectical tension between medical mistrust and trust in Niger. Next I will closely examine mistrust of traditional medicine, Islamic medicine, and biomedicine, considering ways that medical mistrust is embedded in history and in light of the core themes that I have introduced here. I will conclude the chapter by highlighting issues of medical mistrust that crosscut the three major medical sectors.

## Intersecting Precarities and Medical Mistrust in Niger

While Nigériens mistrust all three major medical sectors for different, though often overlapping, reasons, mistrust of health care can generally be linked more broadly to the volatile economic, political, and social conditions in the country. All people live with uncertain futures; however, "intersecting precarities" (MacGregor et al. 2021, 1) and unsettling change are experienced in particularly profound and acute ways in Niger due to a range of contemporary realities. This extreme uncertainty contributes to medical mistrust in Niamey; as Pasquini (2023, 582) observes, "Mistrust [becomes] particularly visible when dealing with situations of great uncertainty."

One of the main ways these precarities manifest themselves in contemporary Niger is through the link between poverty and poor health. Over the last three decades, Niger has been rated at or very near the bottom of the United Nations Human Development Index.[2] In 2021–2022 Niger was rated 189th of 191 nations evaluated because life expectancy at birth is only 61.6 years, the mean years of schooling for those over 25 years is just 2.1 years, and the Gross National Income per capita is only $1,240 (UNDP 2022). Nigérien lives are typically neither long nor healthy. Communicable and nutritional diseases such as diarrheal diseases, malaria, and lower respiratory infections as well as neonatal disorders constitute the leading causes of death in Niger (IHME 2019). Measles and meningitis epidemics plague the country annually, and Nigériens suffer from diseases such as polio and leprosy that have been erad-icated nearly everywhere else in the world. Low life expectancy coupled with the highest fertility rate in the world—7.6 children per woman—means that Niger has the world's youngest population, with a median age of 15 years. Nigériens are aware of their health problems and low life expectancy, issues that signal to them that their medical system is not working and thus contrib-uting to widespread medical mistrust.

These problems are partly due to the fact that Niger's public health system was gutted by a series of structural adjustment programs negotiated with the World Bank and the International Monetary Fund and is chronically under-funded. International and local NGOs have partially filled the gap. This weak system, together with a variety of factors that have led to mistrust of both public and private biomedical facilities, have contributed to people seeking out various forms of healing on their own in the informal sector, through therapy management groups, and reliance on dense social support networks.

The paucity of "human development" in Niger today intersects with other precarities, including violent conflict, climate change, and political upheaval. Violence along Niger's borderlands today, even for Nigériens who have not experienced it firsthand, contributes to increased uncertainty and fear and the inability to move freely. This includes the inability to travel to biomedical clin-ics or village market days when medicines are sold and interferes with heal-ers' ability to visit the bush to collect plant medicines. Niger is surrounded by conflicts and terrorist groups in Nigeria, Libya, Mali, and Burkina Faso that have spilled over its porous borders and led to roughly one million refugees entering the country over the past decade, as well as tens of thousands of inter-nally displaced persons. The Nigeria-based Boko Haram jihadist movement has been menacing people in northeastern Nigeria, southeastern Niger, and western Cameroon for more than a decade through kidnappings and terror-ist attacks on markets, mosques, and schools that have killed roughly 20,000 people. (Nevertheless, Mariama was willing to risk travel into a conflict zone in her quest for healing.) Nigériens living along the borders with Mali and

Burkina Faso have suffered almost daily lethal attacks in the past few years perpetrated by Al Qaeda in the Islamic Maghreb (AQIM), Jamaat Nusrat Al-Islam wal Muslimeen (JNIM), and Islamic State. The influx of refugees has seriously strained the limited resources—including those for medicines—of the Nigérien state and of ordinary families. More than half of these refugees are Nigériens who had been working abroad and sending remittances home to Niger. Roughly half are lodged in refugee camps that are targeted in cross-border raids, while the other half have been absorbed into private compounds—testimony to the remarkable generosity and hospitality of Nigériens.[3]

The deforestation of Niger—due to global warming and reliance of most Nigériens on wood fires for cooking—presents a massive problem for human and environmental health and balance, and a crisis for the health of spirits, many of whom are said to live in trees. Some Nigérien "traditionalists" attribute the multiple crises facing the country to spirits who are angered that they are being neglected and displaced from their homes, and express concern that the loss of trees also means the loss of medicines since all trees are believed to have certain parts (leaves, flowers, bark, roots, etc.) that have healing properties. Similar concerns regarding the loss of spirits' habitat in sacred groves were expressed by the Beng of Côte d'Ivoire (Gottlieb 2008, 250–52). Restricted access to trees due to insecurity, climate change, and poverty fuels mistrust of traditional healers because Nigériens are skeptical that healers have access to all of the best medicines that they could harvest just a decade ago. More broadly, climate change has severely disrupted rainfall patterns in Niger and across the ecologically fragile Sahel, presenting difficult challenges for farmers and herders that have also exacerbated violent conflicts between them in recent years. Thirty-five years ago, when I first visited Niger, the rainy season reliably began at the beginning of June. In recent years, rainy seasons did not begin until July and included more violent storms that have led to large-scale flooding and significant loss of life and property.

In sum, the fragility of health and medical mistrust in Niger are intertwined with the precarious situations described here. That is, Nigériens' willingness to take risks by using multiple kinds of medical systems—despite pervasive mistrust of each of them—can be seen as a logical and reasonable response to intersecting precarities and a quotidian sense of intense uncertainty. In a life full of risks where people most cope with intersecting precarities, many Nigériens make medical decisions even without having confidence in the outcomes. Mistrust can be a practical attitude insofar as it involves seriously assessing other people's intentions and serve as a way of coping with precarious situations of resource shortages (Mühlfried 2019, 33).

## The Dialectical Tension Between
## Mistrust and Trust in Niger[4]

In the afterward of the edited volume *African Medical Pluralism*, influential medical anthropologist Arthur Kleinman (2017, 262) concludes "that the quality of care [in Africa] is increasingly problematic in all forms of caregiving, including those of families, local folk healers, professionalized traditional medical practitioners and biomedical practitioners." Kleinman's general assessment that the quality of caregiving in Africa is in decline in some ways describes what is transpiring in Niamey in particular, as I will describe below. The important point is that many Nigériens perceive that the quality of care and medicines is falling across medical sectors even while therapeutic options are increasing, and this perception fuels medical mistrust.

Nigériens in Niamey are more likely to be isolated from family than they are in rural Niger, where three-quarters of the population lives, because many people in Niamey are newcomers or first- and second-generation migrants. This means they cannot rely as much on family for care and must navigate health systems on their own or with smaller "therapy management groups" than they are accustomed to doing in rural Niger.

Sourcing plant medicines has become increasingly challenging for traditional healers in Niamey, and awareness of this contributes to doubts about their abilities to heal people. Many traditional healers in Niamey do not collect their medicines but purchase them from associates or strangers who have access to the bush. This complicates matters, as most healers in Niamey must trust colleagues to collect medicines and transport them to Niamey, sometimes from hundreds of kilometers away, which also increases their cost. According to my interviews, Nigériens who trust traditional medicine tend to trust traditional healers who gather their own medicines more than those who rely on others, especially others who are not family or close friends, and thus have less confidence in traditional medicine in Niamey than in their rural hometowns and villages. Furthermore, trees and plants that are the primary sources of traditional medicines in Niger are increasingly threatened—as highlighted in my earlier discussion of intersecting precarities—by deforestation, climate change, human settlement expansion, and "terrorists" who have made travel into large areas of the country extremely treacherous. This includes Parc W and its surrounding regions in southwestern Niger that are the most ecologically and medicinally rich areas of the country. Situated just 120 kilometers from and connected to Niamey by one of Niger's few paved roads, this area that has for decades been a crucial source of traditional medicines in the city and is presently cut off from it for the most part.

Islamic medicine is also continuously shifting in Niamey. One of the biggest changes in the last 10 years has been the rise of about 100 men identifying themselves specifically as "Islamic pharmacists" who have opened shops labeled with signage as "Islamic Medicine" pharmacies. Some of these Islamic pharmacists make an effort to publicize their credentials, but most are essentially clerks or vendors who are learning about health and medicine on the fly, partly because a large portion of what they sell is imported and became available only in recent years. In the past, almost all Islamic therapy and medicine in Niamey was provided by local marabouts in their private compounds or at neighborhood mosques that often have small, unmarked shops that sell Islamic literature, prayer beads, and mats alongside a few medicines. Many people in Niamey are wary of these new Islamic pharmacists, the source of their knowledge, their motives, and the nature of their medicines, and yet Islamic pharmacists are proliferating.

In addition, untrained, unlicensed street vendors have emerged over the past 25 years as the most common means of accessing biomedical pharmaceuticals, in part because Niger's public health system has been gutted by neoliberal policies such as structural adjustment programs. Although this practice has grown exponentially primarily due to cost and convenience, many Nigériens also mistrust these vendors and their medicines and are broadly aware of the potential problems associated with the willy-nilly dispensing and consumption of an essentially full range of pharmaceutical drugs.

This snapshot of recent changes in all the major sectors of Niamey is meant to serve as an introduction to a dizzying and ever-changing range of factors that impact how much people trust particular medicines and that they must evaluate in making health related decisions. It is also a reminder that medical mistrust and trust are contextual and constantly shifting.

Nigériens frequently discuss their experience of mistrust of traditional medicine, Islamic medicine, and biomedicine. Indeed, one of the reasons that medical mistrust is so pervasive in Niger is precisely that people regularly discuss it together with family and friends, rather than keeping it to themselves. (The everyday practice of sharing medical mistrust conveniently facilitated

my focus group discussions.) Mistrust, when shared, has "constitutive potential" (Mühlfried 2018, 17) and can serve as a "nexus of sociality, enabling productive ways of interacting with others" (Pasquini 2023, 580). In the Nigérien
case, people depend on family and friends to help them figure out treatment
options precisely because they have low levels of trust in healing professionals. As such, Nigériens form fluid "communities of medical mistrust" involving withholding trust in healers and medicines while actively engaging in
discourse about medical mistrust and how to navigate it.

Nigériens sense that there is a disproportionate share of charlatans among
healers and vendors of medicines in general in Niamey. Only politicians and
state officials are stigmatized as charlatans to the extent that healers are. I am
interested in social perceptions, rumors, and gossip regarding medical mistrust, how patients make decisions in a climate of pervasive suspicion, and the
ways healers navigate the challenges presented by these conditions. I aim to
unravel why it is it that, given Nigériens' widespread mistrust for all options
in the therapeutic landscape of Niamey, they continue to partake not just in
one branch of it, but often all three. In this regard, identifying local understandings of charlatanism and fraud, and recognizing the sources of this local
knowledge, are crucial to refining the analysis. Furthermore, extrapolating
from the theoretical contributions of Mühlfried (2018,11) and Carey (2017,
3) on the dialectical tension between trust and mistrust, I argue that medical
mistrust and trust exist on a continuum in Niger.

At one end of the mistrust–trust spectrum, some Nigériens believe that
certain people posing as healers deliberately harm patients and clients, that
they are the antithesis of healers and are akin to or in fact are predatory sorcerers. Pure charlatans are described by residents of Niamey as people who
willfully offer diagnoses and sell medicines while having no trust in the efficacy of their own products. They are simply in business to make money. At
the opposite end of the mistrust–trust spectrum, many Nigériens have complete trust and confidence in the advice provided by some healers and in the
power of the medicines that they sell. For example, Mariama showed deep
trust in, and was willing to risk her life to visit, a Kanuri healer in Diffa, as
discussed at the opening of the book. A middle-aged Hausa man described
his high level of confidence in the *akwaku* (itinerant pharmaceutical drug
vendors): "We are a poor country and we do not make many things. We rely
on rich countries with high technology to make our lives easier and better by
providing us with cars, cell phones, and pharmaceutical drugs. White people
take these drugs, and they live longer than we do. The *akwaku* sell them at

fair at prices, and they treat me with respect." Most Nigériens express views somewhere in between the polar extremes of complete mistrust and absolute trust of healers. For example, many poor parents are willing to take the risk of purchasing drugs from *akwaku* for their own ailments but choose to drain their savings and borrow money from family and friends to take their children to formal-sector biomedical hospitals, clinics, and pharmacies. Many of my interlocutors indicated that they buy pharmaceuticals on the street for common, simple ailments such as headaches and colds, but visit clinics and pharmacies when they suspect something more serious such as typhoid. Each of these examples reveals partial trust in the *akwaku* as well as a preference for formal-sector biomedical treatments for the most severe ailments. Given their lack of resources, Nigériens sometimes must prioritize who gets what kinds of care. Medical decisions are not based solely on trust but are also significantly influenced and limited by cost and convenience. This is true, on various scales, for most people in the world. Others expressed that they have special trust in a particular healer that they buy medicines from regularly, but none said they only buy from one healer. An elderly Zarma woman's explanation—also regarding the *akwaku*—represents a middle ground that reflects the majority view of the consumers that I interviewed: "We know that the medicines sold by *akwaku* are not as good as those sold in pharmacies, just like we know that the Chinese motorcycles that we ride now are not as good as the Japanese ones that we used to have. But both [street medicines and Chinese motorcycles] work reasonably well and they are what we can afford. I would not keep going to the *akwaku* for drugs if I did not get relief from them. Before, Nigériens could not afford biomedical drugs, but now millions are benefiting from the *akwaku*." The passion expressed regarding healers and medicine is because so much is at stake: These are life-and-death matters.

Anthropologist and cultural theorist Mary Douglas offers useful insights for understanding the complexity of risk—"the probability of an event occurring, combined with the magnitude of the losses or gains that would be entailed" (Douglas 1992, 123). She argues that risk is an inherent part of life because dangers are real. However, not all people are equally vulnerable to dangers or threats to their health. For some people, like many Nigériens, facing chronic health problems is the norm, not the exception. Douglas referred broadly to the reality of danger and risk in "the preindustrial world," but her words aptly capture the realities and uncertainties faced by many people in Niger where there is "low life expectancy . . . mortality rates are high

for everyone . . . [and] starvation, blight, and famine are perennial threats"
(Douglas 1992, 29).

All therapeutic encounters and consumption of medicines are predicated
upon trust and simultaneously involve risks. The fundamental paradox
between trust and risk was identified by social theorist Niklas Luhmann
(1993) who emphasized that one needs to trust someone or something in
order to take certain risks even though trusting someone or something
always carries the risk of disappointment. Furthermore, one might not trust
any healers but might not have any choice but to take a risk, such as trying to
find the healer who one mistrusts the least. Every transaction between healers and their clients entails trust and several kinds of risk for clients. Clients must trust the knowledge and ethics of the healer or at least have trust
in the inherent power of medicines. They also face many risks—knowingly
and unknowingly—including the risk of deception, the risk of losing their
money without getting relief or of becoming sicker, and the risks of error by
the healer or by their own misdiagnoses leading to the purchase of the wrong
kind of medicines or the improper administration of medicines. "Every death
and most illnesses will give scope for defining blameworthiness," as Douglas
(1992, 6) emphasized.

Once they have trust in someone or something, people will continue to
have trust until their expectations are disappointed. In the case of medicine,
this may involve several episodes of disappointment, and even then trust may
endure. In their work in a Hausa-Fulani village in Northern Nigeria 35 years
ago, Etkin et al. (1990, 921, original emphasis) identified a key principle of
Hausa nosology that I found remains consistent among people across ethnic
groups in Niamey today, namely that "The understanding that if a particular medicine fails to effect desired results, this is because it does not 'accept'
(*karba*, meaning also 'receive' or 'befit') the patient, or that the described eti-
ology is in error—*but not that a particular medicine is inherently ineffective*."
Jaffré and Olivier de Sardan (2003) and Sams (2017) have also documented
this perspective in detail. Nigériens continually try new medicines, but do
not discard those that do not seem to work when first used. Rather, they save
them for later use or gift them to family and friends. Just because a certain
medicine did not work for one person does not mean the medicine may not
"accept" and thus heal another person in another situation.

Healers in Niamey face their own sorts of trust issues and risk-taking.
They must trust that their suppliers (plant collectors and wholesale vendors

of Islamic medicine and biomedical pharmaceuticals) are selling them legitimate medicines and offering sound advice. They risk being accused of failing to heal people or worse, making them ill or killing them. A healer that treats someone who later dies may lose clients and may be threatened with violence and feel compelled to move out of the city. Some healers take risks by extending credit to customers. Itinerant pharmaceutical vendors also know that the state could confiscate their goods and shut them down at any point by enforcing existing law that prohibits the sale of pharmaceuticals by unlicensed agents (République du Niger 1997). In the following discussion, I present the different though sometimes overlapping reasons why each health sector—its principles, institutions, healers, and medicines—is viewed with considerable doubt.

## Mistrust of Traditional Medicine in Niger

*The Dangerous Power of Traditional Healers, Even Children.* Patience is a core Nigérien value, but often all bets are off on the roadways where might and wealth make right—trucks have the right of way over buses that have the right of way over cars that have the right way over motorcycles that have the right of way over lowly pedestrians. On a recent, sizzling-hot day in Niamey, a barefoot 10-year-old boy wearing a dirty and tattered t-shirt and football shorts was selling traditional medicine (plant leaves, tree bark, roots, snake skins, and animal bones) from atop a mat on a busy street near the city center. A middle-aged man skidded to a halt on the sand-covered asphalt in his Toyota Corolla just a meter away from the boy, blared his horn, and yelled at the boy to move so that he could park. The boy did not flinch. The man bolted from his car to scream in the boy's face. When the boy calmly responded, "This is my place," the man angrily kicked the boy's medicines onto the sidewalk. As the man turned to walk back to his car, he collapsed in a heap on the road, unable to speak as his body was gripped by violent spasms. This went on for several minutes, and a crowd of curious onlookers gathered. The boy's father returned from an errand and pulled his son aside for a private conversation. Then, the boy walked over to the man, pulled down his trousers, and stuck his finger in the man's rectum. The man's seizures ceased immediately. He pulled up his pants, stood up unsteadily on his feet after the experience, and apologized to the boy and his father. He sheepishly returned to his car and left the scene. I spoke with a few people in the crowd. A Zarma man concluded, "One should never disrespect a traditional healer," and his friend responded, "Not even a child." This extraordinary event illustrates a broader, persistent concern that traditional healers have the power to cure people as well as the power to harm them (Gottlieb 1989; Rasmussen 2001; Stoller 1989; Stoller and Olkes 1987).

Nigériens today express widespread skepticism about traditional medicine and healers, and four reasons for this stand out. First, as highlighted earlier, Pasquini (2023, 580) argued that the healer–patient relationship inherently involves an asymmetry of power that contributes to mistrust. The lingering fear that traditional healers have the power to use poisons and spells to disrupt life plans and cause suffering and death, as illustrated in the vignette, is a dramatic example of mistrust drawn from an unequal power relationship. Second, past and current Islamic movements and narratives have sought to discredit and demonize traditional religions and healers, especially practices involving spirits and spirit possession (Masquelier 2019b), illustrating that medical pluralism contributes to medical mistrust. Third, Nigériens are mistrustful of the accelerating monetization of traditional healing. Fourth, some healers' grandiose claims regarding their abilities to cure all ailments and their spectacular options such as magic money wallets are viewed with widespread doubt.

Muslim Nigériens have suppressed local, traditional religions and their healing practices for centuries (Tremearne 1913), even though for a time parts of Niger were a haven for traditionalists who found refuge from Usman dan Fodio's jihad of 1804 that established the Sokoto Caliphate in northern Nigeria and southwestern Niger (Fuglestad 1983, 24–25). The demonization of traditional religions has accelerated in the last 25 years due to rising Islamist reformist movements that seek to strip away any "African innovations" in Islam (Idrissa 2017; Masquelier 2019b; Sounaye 2013). This suppression is carried out through public preaching and socioeconomic exclusion. Masquelier (2019b, 177–78) describes the iconoclasm of these public performances: "Muslim preachers describe spirits in their sermons as malevolent creatures whose sole aim is to tempt humans into straying from the right path. Spirits, the preachers claim, are Satan's servants, against whom Muslims must guard themselves by relying on the power of prayer. When they attack people, they must be exorcised rather than be allowed to use humans as hosts in the context of ritualized possession performances. And in no circumstances should they be placated through offerings of any kinds, for they are the personification of evil. Having dealings with them is said to lead straight to hell." In short, Muslim preachers and congregations in Niamey have pushed back even further against *Bori* and other local religious practices, especially in the last 15 years. As a result, spirit possession ceremonies in Niamey have been relegated to the margins and are held only late at night, in compounds far away from mosques. Only a handful of possession troupes (spirit praise-singers and musicians) remain in the city, as I mentioned in Chapter 1.

The Nigérien state and its public biomedical health care establishment also work to discredit traditional medicine, even though it permitted l'Association des Tradi-Practiciens du Niger to register as an NGO and nods at the importance of traditional healing by annually observing African Traditional Medicine Day. Periodically Tele-Sahel and Voix du Sahel (state media) report stories of nefarious actions of traditional healers, such as killing children and exhuming graves to harvest organs to be used in magic. I suspect these reports are planted to undermine traditional healers. Regardless, these stories, and permutations of them, circulate widely by word of mouth in Niamey.

The suppression of local traditional religious practices, especially those involving spirit possession, and stories about dreadful traditional healers are linked to the general mistrust of traditional healers and medicines in Niamey. These examples also illustrate that medical pluralism inherently contributes to medical mistrust. Most traditional healers working on the streets of Niamey make no references to spirits or deny that they do when questioned by patients because they are aware of the public mistrust of anything having to do with spirits.

Traditional healers across Niger have always been compensated for their services and medicines, but the accelerating monetization of their profession has damaged their credibility in the minds of some Nigériens. The Tuareg, for example, see a sharp contrast between biomedicine and their traditional medical practices (Rasmussen 2001). Biomedicine is seen as economic medicine or "medicine-for-money" (Rasmussen 2001, 28), whereas Tuareg view their traditional healing as a moral and communal endeavor. This perspective is generally shared across ethnic groups in Niger. One of my participants explained with dismay, "The traditional healers are acting more and more like hospitals and pharmacies—it seems like many are just it in for the money."

In rural Niger, where 75 percent of the population resides, healers are usually known well by their clients. Healers in villages and small towns typically do not ask for specific compensation; rather, they leave it to the patient's discretion, and accept compensation in kind—for example, gifts of grain or livestock (as well as cash). However, some traditional healers require clients to purchase chickens, goats, or cattle, which can be expensive, for use in ritual sacrifice to work with spirits. These patterns are changing throughout Niger, and especially in Niamey and other urban areas where many traditional healers are strangers to their clients, and most demand specific cash payments for medicines and sometimes for consultations. In Chapter 1, I emphasized the central role of rural-to-urban migration in the historical growth of Niamey. Reflecting the demographics of Niamey, many of the people I interviewed, both healers and patients, have within their lifetimes experienced a shift from an intimate, rural setting based on medical sharing and reciprocity to relatively impersonal Niamey where health care and medicine are more thoroughly integrated into the world capitalist economy and care is based on monetary exchange—cash in almost all cases, in such a poor country.[5] In short, many people in Niamey, recent migrants and long-term residents, are mistrustful of traditional healers working on the streets due to the fleeting nature of cash-based interactions with them.

Some Nigériens are turned off by the spectacular claims made by a minority of traditional healers. Many of the traditional healers I interviewed asserted that their knowledge and skills are vastly superior to those of biomedical professionals. Some claim—in person, with professionally painted banners, and online—that they can cure any and all ailments, including AIDS, cancer, and paralysis. Others market virtual panaceas: for example, moringa leaf packaging asserts that it can treat cancer, fatigue, constipation, stomach ulcers, diabetes, hypertension, malaria, inflammation, and mental health as well as serving as an aphrodisiac, smoking cessation tool, and as an appetite enhancer that simultaneously promotes weight loss. Finally, some Nigériens advertise get-rich-quick schemes such as "magic money wallets." The purveyors of these products are not necessarily traditional healers, but in the minds of many Nigériens they are, partly because they use the term "magic" and also because they typically use symbols of traditional divination such as cowrie shells in their marketing, especially online. Various forms of "magic money wallets" are sold in Niger and in many other West African countries. Typically, clients are promised that if they buy a special wallet and vow to do only good things with the money they make from it, then each time clients give money to the magician-vendor, twice as money will appear in the wallet of clients. Magic money wallets can be purchased in person, and money transfers can also be done in person, but more commonly these transactions take place through social media such as WhatsApp and Facebook.

Despite the many factors that contribute to doubt, skepticism, and fear of traditional healers, they remain the most trusted sources for therapy and medicines in Niamey. The insights of Mühlfried (2018, 11) and Pasquini (2023, 580) help resolve this paradox, arguing that mistrust and trust are "mutually constitutive" and rarely absolute. More than 90 percent of the Nigériens I interviewed have used traditional medicine at least once, and some use it exclusively, eschewing Islamic medicine and biomedicine altogether. In many ways traditional health healing principles remain at the base of Nigérien cosmologies and the lens through which Nigériens assess Islamic medicine and biomedicine, as I argued in Chapter 1. The reality is that trust of traditional medicine and healers in Niamey is often contextual and selective rather than absolute. Indeed, Carey (2017, 3) emphasizes that we must specify who or what is trusted, including personal trust in known others, social trust in unknown others, and trust in the "the system"—such as institutions or the state—to appreciate the situational nature of mistrust. For example, my daily observations together with extensive interviews with traditional healers and their clients indicates that "heat" is one of the most common ailments for which patients seek relief, as I discussed at length in Chapter 2. The vast majority of Nigériens in Niger prefer traditional "heat"-specific medicine—a brown plant-infused liquid that is typically served in repurposed drinking water bottles by Nigérienne, Beninoise, and Togolaise women—and do not trust "super-medicines" that are purported to treat "heat" and a long list of other problems. Most Nigériens regard "magic money wallets" and similar ploys as outlandish scams but trust some traditional healers, especially if they know them, and some of the medicines they sell to treat a variety of ailments. Evidently, some Nigériens are attracted by miracle cures, powerful panaceas, and magic money wallets as well as other similar schemes that promise instant cash transfers, or traditional healers and others who claim to have magical powers would not continue to offer them in person and online. Traditional healers are well aware of widespread mistrust of them and make efforts to establish credibility through various strategies such as claiming not to work with spirits, acknowledging their limitations and sometimes referring patients to biomedical care, and occasionally by not requesting specific fees for their services and medicines.

## Mistrust of Islamic Medicine in Niamey

*"What do you know about Islamic medicine?"* In Boukoki, an old neighborhood of Niamey, a group of friends have met daily for 30 years for conversation and to pass the time together on the side of the road under two old neem trees that provide shade most of the day. The group's core figure, Djibrilla, ran a small open-air business selling produce, kola nuts, cigarettes, and cold sodas and provided a few benches and mats for his friends and customers. One day, Elhadji Lamine, the imam of the mosque across the street, informed Djibrilla and the group that he had purchased the compound situated behind the neem trees, and then resold it to a Saudi Arabian NGO that planned to open a guesthouse for traveling Islamic scholars. Djibrilla and company were initially pleased by this turn of events, as the unfriendly family that had lived in the compound with a snarling dog was being replaced by a sort of sacred space occupied by learned men doing charitable work.

A few months later, a Nigérien representative of the NGO informed Djibrilla and his friends that they would need to move because he was going to cut down the two neem trees to create space to build an Islamic medicine shop. Djibrilla was outraged. He yelled at the man, "This is an injustice. What do you know about Islamic medicine? Allah created all trees and put medicinal properties in all of them. No trees should be killed." Elhadji Lamine heard the commotion and came over to intervene. Djibrilla repeated his complaint but relented when Elhadji explained, "This is his property now, and he can do whatever he wants with it." Djibrilla and his friends realized they were powerless to stop the cutting of the trees. They were not happy about it and framed their displeasure in ways that went beyond losing their meeting and business space. They emphasized the importance of trees for community health. Furthermore, they questioned why an NGO was going to open a for-profit business selling medicine. When the store opened, I purchased a box of Add-awa'ul Bawasur medicine produced by the Al-Noor Islamic Health Center in Kano, Nigeria, to establish rapport with the proprietor and to study the packaging. After I read its label that indicates that it treats typhoid, chronic pile, gonorrhea, syphilis, staphylococcus, worms, back pain, and stomach pain to Djibrilla, he laughed and said, "What a ridiculous scam, there is no way that one medicine could treat all of those things."

This series of events and discourse illustrates many core themes regarding doubt about Islamic medicine in Niamey, including disputes about what Islamic medicine is, contestations over social justice, the monetization of

Islamic medicine, and the questioning of quasi-panaceas. It also emphasizes the importance of trees as sources of medicine and the concept of community health, again illustrating the prevalence and importance of traditional medicines in this place.

*The Islamic Pharmacist Charlatan.* In July 2021 I was sitting and chatting with two old friends (Moussa and Rabé) and Issaka, a specialist in Islamic medicine, on benches in the shade outside of Issaka's shop in the Nouveau Marché neighborhood. I asked Issaka, "Do you have medicine for COVID-19?" At the time, no reliable biomedical medication for COVID-19 was yet available, and I was curious to see how he would answer. He responded affirmatively, went into his shop, returned with one of his common shrink-wrapped, industrially labeled, anti-evil spirit medications, and asked 15,000 CFA for it. I studied the label and saw no references to the coronavirus. Meanwhile, Rabé took a walk down the block. Moussa asked me to call Rabé. When I did, Rabé warned me not to buy the exorbitantly priced medicine and emphasized, "There are no cures for COVID-19, and we are not even sure that it exists." I politely declined to purchase the medicine.

This incident led me to experience doubt about the integrity of this Islamic healer. Not only did Issaka quintuple his normal asking price—in the recent past I bought several boxes of very similar medicines for 3,000 FCFA or less from him—but he was willing to treat an illness that he may not believe even exists. Rabé's comments also reflect the widespread skepticism expressed by Nigériens regarding mass biomedical messaging and vaccination campaigns.

Ninety-eight percent of Nigériens are Muslim (Idrissa 2020, 285) who trust in God and share the belief that faith, prayer, and fasting are obligatory and are necessary for physical, spiritual, and emotional well-being. Beyond that, Nigériens vary considerably in their trust in Islamic medicine, ranging from people who use it exclusively to others who beyond daily prayers and fasting during Ramadan visit only traditional or biomedical healers or both.

Islam and Islamic medicine have never been uniformly practiced or static in Niger. However, as I discussed in Chapter 1, over the last 30 years and especially in the last decade, definitions of proper Muslim belief and practice have been and continue to be increasingly contested, debated, and shifting. In short, conservative Salafist movements originating in Saudi Arabia have become more and more influential in Niger, first indirectly through groups that they had influenced in Northern Nigeria, and more recently through direct religious investment in Niger and growing numbers of Nigérien students who are training in Islamic universities in Saudi Arabia and returning to lead mosques and deliver sermons in Niger. Salafist preachers have denounced mainstream, traditional Sunni Islam as well as Sufi Islam just as vehemently as they have denounced traditional Nigérien religions, if not more so. This includes local healing practices. Influential preacher Elhadji Mamane expressed the increasingly common position that: "The only people worse than animists who play with African spirits are ignorant hypocrites who mix Islam and animist practice." Many Nigériens, especially those who came of age before this fundamentalist turn, feel confused or insulted by these attacks on their belief and practice.

Medical mistrust is situationally variable, can shift over time (Sengul and Bulut 2020, 1232), and emerges particularly in times of uncertainty (Mühlfried 2018, 11). The contemporary unsettled moment in Niger that has led to ambiguity and debates about what exactly Islamic medicine is as well as to debates about what forms of non-Islamic healing are permissible for Muslims to use illustrates these theoretical insights. "Islamic medicine" can be defined as the set of principles and practices of health and healing articulated in the Qur'an and the Hadiths as well as the wide variety of ideas and practices Muslim people absorbed from various cultures, as I discussed in the previous chapter. These include practices and medicines that are used both prophylactically or to treat existing ailments, such as prayer, drinking chalk from Qur'anic slates, holy water, fasting, honey and other "food-medicines," and the writing of Qur'anic texts on pieces of paper that are sometimes folded and inserted and sewn into leather amulets worn on the body. Since only a minority of Nigériens can read and understand the Qur'an and the Hadiths, most Nigériens rely on imams and preachers to inform them about what Islamic medicine is and what forms of traditional medicine and biomedicine are acceptable.[6] In traditional practice, some of these amulets are filled with plant medicine and have been denounced by some preachers as African innovations that are contrary to Islam. In everyday practice, Islamic medicine is what people say it is. Some Nigérien Islamic scholars have more authority and capacity to reach large audiences than others through public sermons, CD recordings, and television appearances, but their narratives vary regarding Islamic medicine and the forms of traditional medicine and biomedicine that are acceptable for proper Muslims (Sounaye 2013). Many Nigériens fully trust only one imam (at a time) and only one Islamic healer that they know and are wary to various extents about others. This is all fluid because individual imams change their perspectives, some imams lose popularity,

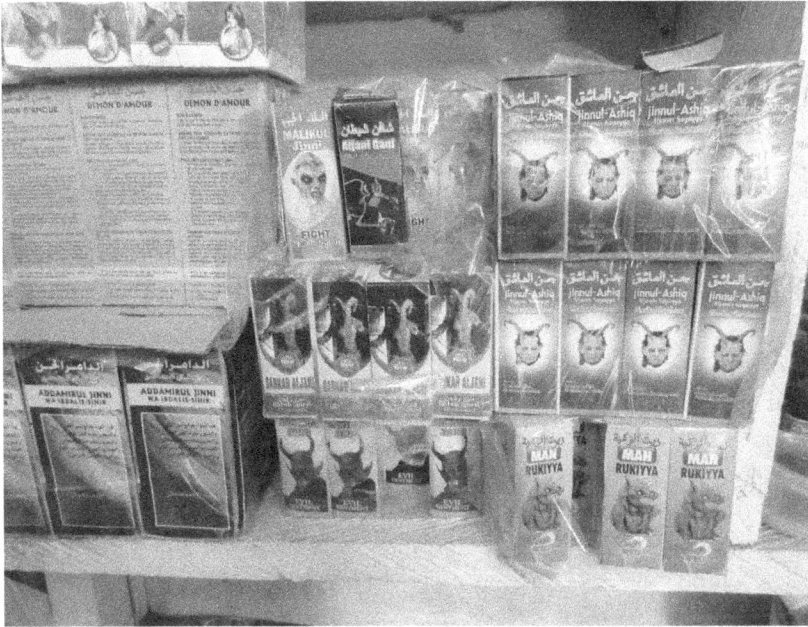

Figure 3.1. Islamic anti-evil spirit medicine. Photo by author.

and new imams emerge with regularity. Furthermore, new and controversial forms of imported Islamic medicine have become available in Islamic medicine shops and on the streets of Niamey in the last few years.

My earlier discussion of factors leading to mistrust of traditional medicine highlighted Muslim preachers' attacks on spirits and on people who seek to communicate with or appease spirits through possession and sacrifice. In contrast, some Nigérien Muslims think that Islamic medicine does not know how to deal effectively with local spirits—that the Islamic strategies of forcefully exorcising spirits can never fully work and can backfire and intensify the anger of spirits. Most of the medicine sold in Islamic medicine shops of Niamey is made in Northern Nigeria to repel attacks by witches, sorcerers, demons, zombies, and evil spirits, or to exorcise malicious spirits. The labeling of these medicines typically includes Arabic, Hausa, and English descriptions, borrows ideas from biomedical packaging, and draws liberally from global horror film imagery. Most Nigériens that I interviewed about it do not know what to make of it. In a focus group discussion of middle-aged Hausa men, one explained, "We do not know what is in it [packaged Islamic medicine] because the ingredients are never listed." His friend wondered, "Is it even Islamic medicine?" Another man similarly asked, "What makes it Islamic medicine?" His associate responded, "They want us to believe that if it was made by an Islamic pharmacist and has Arabic on the label, then it must be Islamic medicine. But we know that anyone can put anything they want on a label." His friend added, "Our imam teaches witches and zombies and the like do not exist, that they are just superstitions." No one in this group of eight men was willing to purchase any of this new Islamic medicine, but most said that they would be willing to try it if someone gave it to them. I purchased many boxes of this new Islamic medicine to study the labels, and I had no trouble finding friends and workers in the compound where I was staying who were happy to try it. The high value on gift-giving in Niger explains why many Nigériens are willing to try medicines that they are unwilling to purchase. In Niger, gift-giving is more than a way of solidifying social relationships through reciprocity (Mauss 1954), it is vital to the survival of millions of people in one of the world's poorest countries. Healing in Niamey is often a community matter shaped by social relations (Carey 2017) and "therapy management groups" (Janzen 1978). Aside from skepticism about some of the new forms of Islamic medicine in Niamey, criticism of Islamic medicine by traditional and biomedical healers is muted.


## Mistrust of Biomedicine in Niger

*Sciatic Nerve Injuries Due to Clinical Error.* A tragically high percentage of Nigériens in Niamey suffer from paralysis of one or both legs—at probably a higher rate than any other place in the world except for some war and postwar zones. Some lead economically productive lives, are married with children, and are happy, but many more lead very difficult lives in a country where little is done to accommodate people with disabilities. Many Nigériens who have lost the use of one or both legs survive by begging while moving on the streets of Niamey with crutches, wheelchairs, skateboards and, for the very poorest, by crawling. I think there are three main causes of lower limb paralysis in Niger. Some are due to broken bones that were not set properly, either by traditional bonesetters or by physicians. Paralysis is also a symptom of polio that remains endemic in Niger, typically affecting both legs but sometimes only one. Many suffer from sciatic nerve injuries—usually to the peroneal nerve, a branch of the sciatic nerve—caused by botched administrations of vaccinations in their buttocks. The latter injury is associated with biomedicine, since vaccines are typically administered in public health clinics.

I suspect—drawing from interviews and informal conversations—that vaccination-induced sciatic nerve injuries may be the leading cause of leg paralysis in Niamey. I was unable to locate any research on the subject in Niger, but many studies in Nigeria, especially Northern Nigeria, document that it is a significant public health problem there (Fatunde and Familusi 2001; Idowu et al. 2011). My research offers a few clues, though it is incomplete. For one thing, it is nearly impossible to visually differentiate between a leg stricken by polio and one maimed by a syringe. For another thing, I felt uncomfortable asking people with disabilities questions about their disability due to my own inclinations as well as my awareness that it can be a sensitive topic among Nigériens. Vaccination-induced sciatic nerve injuries can be excruciatingly painful from the point of contact with the needle to many years of chronic, debilitating pain. In my conversations with a few people with the condition whom I know well, they indicated that over time the afflicted leg becomes numb. In many cases the leg muscles completely wither away and/or drop foot develops, a condition wherein the foot "drops" or becomes twisted, sometimes by 180 degrees.

Several generations of Nigériens have suffered from this "stupid," easily avoidable injury caused by clinical ineptitude (Farmer 2010). I have never heard of any organized protests regarding this problem. However, Mohammadou, a good friend who lost the use of left leg due to a childhood injection that went awry, explained to me, "I am not bitter or angry about what happened to me. Patience is the key to life and sanity. Allah protects me, amen." Then, he added a Hausa proverb that is best figuratively translated as "Fool me once, shame on you, fool me twice, shame on me." By this, he continued, he meant that he will never go to biomedical facility again in his life. I think this is a typical perspective. However, I know others with the condition who regularly use pharmaceutical drugs.

Vaccination-induced sciatic nerve injuries contribute significantly to mistrust of syringes, vaccinations, and biomedicine in general in Niamey. Their ubiquity in Niamey serves as a daily visual reminder of, and warning about the dangers of biomedicine. Almost everyone in Niamey personally knows someone who suffered the injury and sees many people daily who did. Reflecting global patterns (Boyas and Valera 2011, 145), educated and wealthy Nigériens are more likely than uneducated and poor Nigériens to seek vaccinations than poor Nigériens, which in some ways makes the educated more vulnerable than the uneducated to sciatic injuries. However, wealthy Nigériens are more likely to have access to competent health care workers in the private clinics than the poor are in public clinics. Hence, it is a problem that impacts people across class lines.

Many scholars have emphasized that "The legitimacy of medical scientific 'truth,' particularly within the context of Western medicine, has always been tenuous in Africa" (Ogala 2021, 308). In the minds of some Nigériens, biomedicine is tainted by its real and perceived association with colonialism, racism and Islamophobia, France, the West, and a corrupt Nigérien state. Nevertheless, biomedical care is central to the therapeutic itineraries of millions of Nigériens. That is, it is not necessarily biomedicine per se that is mistrusted by Nigériens. Rather, it is a host of other issues associated with biomedicine that are mistrusted, such as its impersonal mode of delivery, high costs, low quality of care, a sense that mass public health campaigns focus on the wrong problems rather than more pressing health concerns, and its association with the state in general and its public health policies. Mistrust of biomedicine in Niger is also connected to more recent historical developments and large-scale public health initiatives.

The collapse of the Soviet Union and the ostensible end to the Cold War gave the U.S. and the West added leverage to push African countries to enact political, economic, and public health reforms as a condition for continuing aid and foreign direct investment. Between 1990 and 1993, nine Francophone African countries and several others convened National Conferences that initiated the transition from single-party rule to multiparty electoral democracies and promoted neoliberal economic reforms. Niger held its National Conference from July to November 1991. The "democracy era" of multiparty elections that followed the National Conference led to accelerating Western influence on health policies in Niger, including increasing privatization and "NGO-ization" of biomedical healthcare services.

Through the 1980s, very few African presidents considered family planning or population growth to be an important issue or found it too risky to discuss, "A striking exception was a speech made in Matameye [Niger] in 1985 by the late President of Niger Seyni Kountché, who stressed the huge demographic challenge confronting Niger" (Barrère et al. 1999, 3, cited in May 2016, 314). During and immediately after Niger's political-economic transformation, the first two health initiatives in sequence pushed in Niger by Western governmental and especially non-governmental organizations with the tepid support of the Nigérien state were family planning and polio vaccinations. These included the U.S. Agency for International Development (USAID), United Nations Population Fund (UNPF), CARE, and Save the Children, among others (Cooper 2019). Shortly after these initial steps, public and private health messaging shifted by including the promotion of condom use as a means of preventing the spread of HIV and AIDS. I recall from visits in the 1990s that many Nigériens were puzzled. As a friend put it, "We are not sure what the West wants. On the one hand, they want us to limit our population. On the other hand, they want us to have sex with anyone."

Family planning and condom use were and are widely regarded as nefarious plots designed to undermine traditional Nigérien values and to sterilize and thus control African Muslims. For most Nigériens, infertility is a far greater concern than limiting family sizes (Cooper 2019; Moussa 2023). Polio vaccination campaigns were sometimes viewed as part of the same global conspiracy in many communities of southern Niger (Cooper 2019; Masquelier 2012) and Northern Nigeria (Renne 2010). This conclusion draws from the reality that the mass campaign to eradicate polio was initiated virtually simultaneously with family planning and AIDS policies, as well as widespread local knowledge of counterfeit meningitis vaccines administered in Niger and a catastrophic trial of an experimental meningitis vaccine in nearby Northern Nigeria, both in the 1990s (Archibong and Annan 2021; Sams and Hrynick 2020, 20). As Sams and Hrynick (2020, 20) emphasize, resistance to oral polio vaccines (OPV) in parts of southern Niger was much more than "a matter of religious refusal or simple ignorance [but] actually a much more complex story in which several factors interacted with and reinforced one another. First, people were put off by abrupt health workers . . . [and knew that] counterfeit meningitis vaccines administered in Niger in the 1990s had also allegedly killed thousands of children. Secondly, people were suspicious of the considerable resources put towards the OPV campaign (with health workers visiting every home) as they had only ever experienced a barely functioning health system." Many Nigériens who questioned the focus on polio because so many diseases kill many more people now question the focus on COVID-19 for the same reasons (Sams and Hrynick 2020). This crisis-driven approach makes little sense to Nigériens who do not perceive that COVID-19 is a crisis. Nigériens understand that COVID-19 is a crisis in other parts of the world but are much more concerned about diseases like malaria that directly threaten their day-to-day health. Most Nigériens do not wholly mistrust biomedicine. However, as these examples show, Nigériens are highly mistrustful of public health initiatives—family planning, HIV-AIDS prevention, polio and COVID-19 vaccinations—originating in the West. It is not just that these policies are foreign; to many Nigériens they address the wrong problems—or as in the case of family planning, issues that are not perceived as problems.

Formal-sector biomedical hospitals, clinics, pharmacies, physicians, and pharmacists terrify many Nigériens due to problems documented by many scholars, including shortages of medicine; long waiting times for patients; clinical negligence due to the carelessness, inexperience, and incompetence of health care workers; the flagrant cruelty of health care workers who demand bribes for referrals and to complete procedures that they have initiated; and discrimination against the poor (Cooper 2019; Heller 2019; Jaffré and Olivier de Sardan 2003; Rasmussen 2001). Formal sector health professionals in Niamey are typically strangers to their clients and frequently—though not always—treat patients rudely; for example, by only using French with non-French speaking clients, even when they know local languages. Gottlieb (2004) documented that this practice is also common in Côte d'Ivoire. This use of a language that signifies the providers' education and distances less formally educated patients is a mark of what Pasquini (2023) highlights as an inherently asymmetrical relationship between healers and patients, which involves a disparity of knowledge and power. While such disparities can certainly lead to mistrust, they rarely lead to the collapse of health-care interactions. Instead, patients and providers experience "mistrustful dependency," meaning that "mistrust manifests as risk management strategies in asymmetric care relationships" (Pasquini 2023, 588–89). For Nigérien patients, then, mistrust partly springs out of the unequal relationships they find themselves in with biomedical providers (and, indeed, other healers), but this mistrust can prove to be a useful tool in navigating these systems.

Furthermore, as a strategy to build national unity and to combat corruption, the Nigérien state has for decades moved civil servants—including health care workers—far from their home regions. This has led to significant social ruptures and increases mistrust of health care personnel (Olivier de Sardan 2006, Sams 2021). Language barriers and "ethnic discordance" between health care workers and patients lead to mistrust of health care workers, especially when the former represent a majority group and the latter a minority group. This issue has also been documented extensively in the U.S. (Boyas and Valera 2011). The extremity of Niger's poverty does not make it a unique case of medical mistrust.

Traditional healers and Islamic healers criticize biomedicine as foreign and thus ill-suited for Nigériens and because it uses harmful artificial chemicals, contributing to the mistrust of biomedicine. In contrast, they consistently promote their services as proper for Nigériens because their medicines draw on local cultural heritage and are "natural," "plant-based," and "organic." Some traditional and Islamic healers also argue that some biomedical practices and policies—such as contraception, abortion, and mandatory vaccinations—violate local cultural and religious values. In turn, formal-sector biomedical professionals warn Nigériens of the hazards of traditional medicine, Islamic medicine, and the biomedical pharmaceuticals sold by unregulated street healers in the informal sector. They do so in a variety of ways, including through public service announcements on radio stations and billboards, labels on pharmacy bags warning patients of the dangers of street medicines, and by verbally imploring clients to stay away from all informal-sector healers.

In the only known research on the quality of pharmaceuticals sold on the street in Niamey, Pouillot et al. (2008, 17) found that 26 of 45 pharmaceuticals tested did not conform to package label claims. A wide variety of local and international media have reported on Nigérien radio stations and websites the importation or manufacturing of fake, counterfeit, and illicit drugs in Niger (iciniger.com 2018; Niamey.com 2017; Observer 2018). Although relatively few Nigériens read these stories, those who do share them, and they have become part of everyday discussion and rumor, casting a shadow of uncertainty on pharmaceutical drugs in Niamey's informal sector. Medical pluralism and competition for clients between medical sectors fuels medical mistrust.

However, I heard a consistent refrain in my interviews and conversations with formal-sector health care professionals as well as among patients who trust only biomedicine. That is, many think that some traditional and Islamic plant medicines probably have some healing properties, but because traditional and Islamic healers have no formal scientific training, they have no idea about proper dosages or of possible interactions of plant medicines with other plant medicines or with pharmaceuticals, and thus can harm or kill patients.

Despite their reasons for mistrusting biomedicine, biomedicine is a crucially important in the health care of Nigériens. Today in Niamey, most parents choose a standard course of vaccinations for their children. For example, in Niger the percentage of surviving infants who received the third dose of DTP-containing vaccine rose from 6 percent in 1981 to 84 percent in

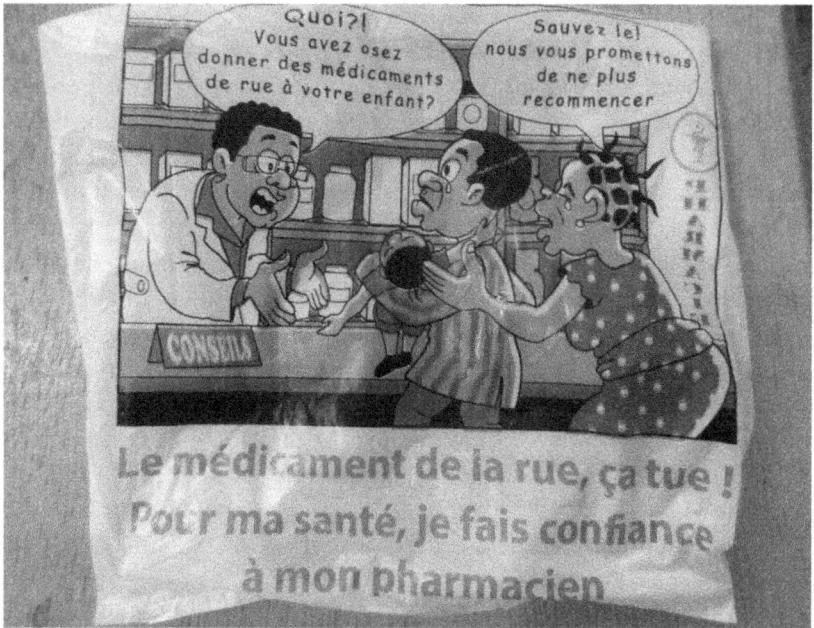

Figure 3.2. Formal-sector pharmacy bag. (Translation of bottom caption: "Street Medicine Kills! For my health, I trust my pharmacist.") Photo by author.

2022 (UNICEF 2023). Indeed, vaccine avoidance is highly contextual, "For instance, thanks to vaccination campaigns, the administrative estimate of vaccine coverage in the 2021 meningitis outbreak zone (Niamey) was 85%, and in the 2021 cholera outbreak zone (Maradi) 92%" (WHO 2021). These examples reveal the complexity of contextual medical mistrust because they occurred simultaneously with the rejection COVID-19 vaccinations by almost all Nigériens. Indeed, after more than three years of the pandemic, as of July 30, 2023, only 23.8 percent of Nigériens had received at least one dose of the COVID-19 vaccine (Our World in Data 2023).

Most people in Niamey choose to go to hospitals for their most serious ailments, even if it is not their first choice. Just as anthropologists Mühlfried (2018) and Carey (2017) broadly theorized, mistrust of biomedicine is usually not absolute among Nigériens but contextual. Much of the mistrust of biomedicine is directed toward formal-sector institutions and practitioners as well as the state and global institutions such as the WHO and their emergency health policies. In contrast, surging numbers of Nigériens over the past

25 years have come to rely on pharmaceutical drugs sold by mobile street vendors. Many Nigériens regard street biomedicine as fundamentally different from formal-sector biomedicine due to the former's much lower prices and convenience, and the narrow social distances between healers and patients.

## Conclusion

In this chapter, I have argued that grappling with medical mistrust is an everyday concern for millions of Nigériens. I have shown Nigériens do not need complete trust to make therapeutic decisions, that in fact they rarely fully trust the healers they visit or their medicines. They act, they find options—including electing to forgo certain vaccinations at particular times—that make them think and feel that they are minimizing risks in a context of worry that some healers and some healing institutions are determined to kill them. I also emphasized that medical mistrust is context-dependent in many ways and included multiple examples.

The medical mistrust–trust nexus is universal, though it manifests itself in different ways around the world. The following summary of key variables influencing medical mistrust and trust across all medical sectors in Niger may therefore also offer useful insights for understanding mistrust and trust in many countries, including the U.S., as well as providing context for understanding how Nigériens navigate the proverbial minefield of medical mistrust as discussed in the following chapter. In Niger, four factors impacting the mistrust–trust continuum stand out above others: the particular dynamics of medical pluralism, the relative newness of healers and medicines, social identities, and social and power distances. Each of these variables is extremely fluid. Therefore, I am not proposing that they can be used to reliably predict Nigériens' medical decisions before they make them.

Because three medical sectors share, roughly equally, the therapeutic landscape in Niger, representatives, healers, and proponents of each sector actively work to discredit the principles, healers, and medicines of other sectors, contributing to mistrust. In "theory" it does not need to be this way. The three sectors could work harmoniously together rather than competitively, and sometimes they do, as some healers share knowledge and refer clients across medical sectors in Niger.

Nigériens sometimes find certain new medicines from particular places, such as Islamic medicine made in Saudi Arabia, very appealing, as I showed in Chapter 1. In contrast, in this chapter I have emphasized that Nigériens approach new types of healers and medicines with great caution and skepticism. However, this does not stop some Nigériens from experimenting with new healers and medicines if they are convenient or affordable or if family and friends have gifted medicines to them.

Social identities in Niger can impact which healers and medicines people mistrust or trust. Traditional-localist, Muslim, and modern-Francophone constitute the three main social identities in Niger (R. Idrissa 2021, Sams 2017, Youngstedt 2013). This, of course, is a rough generalization, partly because these identities are often contextual in Niger. Furthermore, millions of Nigériens see these three sorts of identities as complementary and not as mutually exclusive. There are nevertheless some Nigériens who emphasize one of these three models as their core identity, and in interviews and focus groups they reported being more likely to trust the healers and medicines associated with the core identity than those of other sectors, and more likely to mistrust and denigrate medical sectors outside of the one they trust most. However, many exceptions show how loose the generalization is. I encountered a substantial minority of highly educated Nigériens—in the Franco-Nigérien secular sense of the word "education"—who trust traditional medicine more than biomedicine, including some who use traditional medicine exclusively, as well as many uneducated people who trust biomedicine far more than they trust traditional or Islamic medicine. Furthermore, many Nigériens across all three identity constructions regularly mix-and-match therapies across medical sectors, for example by using traditional medicine to treat heat–cold, Islamic medicine such as *miel coranisée* (French for Qur'anicized or sacred honey) on cuts and scrapes, and biomedicine such as vaccinations.

Social distances and power distances are crucial variables in the mistrust–trust nexus in Niger and in many other places. In general, Nigérien patients strongly prefer the narrowest possible social and power distances (in terms of ethnicity, class, and gender) between themselves and healers and health institutions. However, which if any of these variables comes to forefront depends on particular contexts. Women strongly prefer traditional women healers over other healers for female-specific challenges, such as fertility, pregnancy, and childbirth. Mariama, a Hausa woman, sought treatment from a Kanuri man, showing that sometimes the reputation of a famous healer can trump ethnicity and gender. A Zarma patient is more likely to trust a Hausa street vendor of pharmaceutical drugs who is his neighbor and of comparable socioeconomic means and treats him with respect in Zarma over a formal-sector

Zarma biomedical professional who is a wealthier stranger who treats him with disrespect and speaks to him in French. Furthermore, the mistrust of the commodification of medicines, especially the high costs of formal-sector biomedicine, can be seen as a dimension of power distances between healers and patients.

Nigériens regularly work to disrupt power distance hierarchies between themselves and healers. Denigrating traditional healers for working with spirits, Islamic pharmacists for their perceived lack of knowledge of their own products, and biomedical physicians for their corruption serve as challenges to asymmetric care relationships and ways of diminishing the reputations of healers. In Niger, medical mistrust functions as an attitude of rugged-autonomy-in-community that meshes neatly with the prevalence of self-care and therapy management groups and the general ethos in Niamey that everyone is a healer of sorts, as described in Chapter 1, and can serve as a useful attitude for navigating intersecting precarities.

## CHAPTER 4

# Navigating Medical Mistrust and Medical Pluralism in Niger

I n this chapter, I will focus on analyzing the ways Nigériens navigate options within and between traditional, Islamic, biomedical sectors both sequentially and simultaneously despite pervasive mistrust of each sector. Following the lead of anthropologists Sargent and Kennell (2017, 241), "In seeking to understand suffering as patients follow an elusive path to health, we might benefit from asking 'What options when, and why?' 'What external forces determine the fluidity of options?' and 'What makes a particular option untenable?'" These questions are valuable to consider, and I assert that answers to these questions are best illustrated through discussion and analysis of specific illnesses and therapeutic experiences of individual Nigériens. I also argue that in answering them, it is critical to pay attention to the attitudes and beliefs that guide patients' decision-making. In this case, pervasive mistrust shapes most Nigériens' medical choices and experiences. Hence, much of this chapter is devoted to two case studies. The first involves a group of five men—a father, his son, and three friends—and the medical decisions they made alone and together as each faced illnesses of varying degrees of severity. The second focuses on the "health life history" of one man. In addition, I draw from extensive interview and focus group data on these and similar questions to broaden the analysis.

The use of biomedicine is ascending, as highlighted in my discussion of the history of medical pluralism in Niger in Chapter 1. However, as in much of Africa (Janzen 2017, 90), the rise of biomedicine in Niger has not led to a decline in the use of traditional medicine or Islamic medicine. Local spirits, sorcerers, witches, and "ethno-maladies" (Taylor 2017, 181) such as heat–cold remain real for many Nigériens, including those with advanced scientific training. Put another way, while they have had to adapt to an expanding and competitive therapeutic landscape, traditional and Islamic healers are neither going out of business nor losing significant numbers of clients as a result of the popularity of biomedicine. Instead, an ever-increasing range of options are (potentially) available to Nigériens. This is not unique to Niger. Schoepf (2017, 111) argues that across African contexts, "Amazing bricolages, inventively hybrid combinations of divination, herbal medicines, and spirit mediumship are buttressed by paraphernalia, disease categories, terminology, and medications derived from biomedicine." However, while Nigériens appreciate having therapeutic options, the very existence of three constantly changing major medical sectors fuels medical mistrust. Many Nigériens conclude that all three medical sectors cannot be valid, in part because healers of each sector work to discredit healers and medicines of other sectors.

Nigériens find it difficult to know which healers and which medicines to trust in part because of continuities and discontinuities in each medical sector. Recall the significant changes in each sector over the past 25 years. Traditional medicine is increasingly imported from places near and far and packaged, and healers established a multiethnic association to promote their profession. The Islamic medical landscape has expanded with an increasing number of men identifying themselves as Islamic pharmacists who offer packaged medicines imported from Saudi Arabia and other Arab countries, as well as Nigeria, India, Pakistan, and Indonesia. The emergence of the *akwaku*, mobile pharmaceutical vendors, has significantly accelerated access to biomedicine. In each case, Nigériens are simultaneously curious about and mistrustful of new options. I found that many people are too mistrustful initially to purchase new medicines for themselves but are curious enough to try them when they are gifted to them by family or friends.

Masquelier (2019, 203) emphasizes that Nigériens "zigzag" through life, negotiating "uncertain economic contexts by broadening their repertoire of income-earning activities, adapting to changing conditions, and engaging in incessant hustle." Many Nigériens work as motorcycle mechanics one month, as mango vendors the next, and as street pharmaceutical vendors the following month. Nigériens' relentless healing quests often involve zigzagging through multiple healing modalities, sequentially or simultaneously, depending on their means, beliefs, and social identities. Ninety percent of the hundreds of Nigériens that I interviewed and conversed with have sought or continue to seek therapy from each of the three main sectors of medicine in Niamey—plant medicine and spiritual therapy, Islamic medicine, and biomedicine. Many explained that they simultaneously take biomedical and plant remedies, especially if they are unsure of the origin of their ailments. Many others start with one healing regimen, often inspired by social identities, but will switch to another one if the first fails to provide relief. Nigériens also recognize that many illnesses and vulnerable health conditions such as pregnancy entail a progression of symptoms that must be treated with a progression of therapies within or between medical sectors. Heat–cold is another example, as it may begin with internal symptoms such as stomach bloating that are treated with various medicines before it externalizes itself through acne or skin blotches that require entirely different treatments. Sargent and Kennell (2017, 227) offer a parallel argument that warrants a lengthy citation because it applies to medical decision-making in Niger,

> Our ethnographic research [in Benin], and that of others [in various African countries] . . . suggests that patients, often with the advice of kin and friends, consult diverse practitioners as diagnoses evolve over time, as efficacy of treatments waxes and wanes, as symptoms are interpreted and reinterpreted, and as new counsel is offered by respected others. Consulting an herbalist, a ritual specialist, an evangelical preacher [or Muslim scholar], and a physician for the same illness episode may seem incompatible, if not contradictory, acts. Yet from the patient's perspective, these may be initiatives drawn from a field of possibilities, not necessarily in epistemological competition, but rather, appropriate at a given moment in an illness trajectory.

Last (1981) similarly argues that the pursuit of health among Hausa across the spectrum of medical pluralism involves pragmatic and flexible reasoning, which is analogous to the flexible, progressive approaches to healing highlighted by Sargent and Kennell (2017) and the "zigzagging" in everyday life identified by Masquelier (2019).

Therapeutic eclecticism is the norm throughout Africa (Olsen and Sargent 2017). For example, in his study of cancer care in Kenyan hospital ward, Mulemi (2017, 220, 223) found that "Patients want the opportunity to exercise self-directing freedom to enhance well-being, drawing on available resources and the care community. An important dimension to this is the right of patients to information on his or her disease and alternative treatment options . . . patients prefer different therapies in a complementary fashion, rather than in isolation." By "different therapies" Mulemi is referring to the use of traditional medicine among patients while they are in a cancer ward. These "alternative options" are provided by family and friends during visits, not dispensed by the hospital. In my discussion of the supportive care provided by therapy management groups in Niger in the Introduction, I noted that one dimension of this assistance is providing meals for patients staying in public hospitals. When I joined groups that were visiting hospitalized family and friends, I also observed that care communities discreetly gave patients packets of traditional medicine or had cooked it into the meals they brought with them from home. They explained that hospital staff discouraged this but did little to prevent it. Nigérien patients like to have access to as many therapeutic options as possible. Since they widely mistrust healers and medicines, the more options they have the more likely they are to find one that they do trust or at least mistrust less than other choices.

Nigériens in general share with Kenyan cancer patients a desire for autonomy in medical decision-making. Indeed, in the Introduction I emphasized the centrality of self-care in the context of "therapy management groups" and noted that many Nigériens to some degree consider themselves as healers. The preference for medical pluralism among Nigérien patients makes sense in this context. However, despite the strong preference for self-autonomy, Nigériens rely on street healers in each medical sector for, if nothing else, obtaining the ingredients for creating their own home-based remedies. Roberts's (2021, 10) discussion of the therapeutic landscape in Accra, Ghana, also serves as an accurate description of Niamey, "The city has an open healing culture, one that has appropriated healing ideas, practices, and goods from both African and Atlantic [and Asian] circuits . . . This means that a sufferer must shop their sickness around, seeking help from as many people as possible to find a cure." Many Nigériens do not regard traditional, Islamic, and biomedical therapies as distinct, but rather as overlapping. Among countless examples of these medical intersections, I will highlight a few prominent, recurring themes. Many Nigériens rely on biomedical diagnoses of their illnesses and treat them with traditional medicines either because they mistrust pharmaceutical drugs or because they cannot afford them. Some healers of each sector refer patients to healers of other sectors. Patients may use biomedicine for symptom relief of their ailments while consulting with traditional herbalists or diviners to find the underlying causes of their suffering, especially when they suspect supernatural involvement. Akin to what Sargent and Kennell (2017, 241, emphasis added) found in neighboring Benin,

"These cases suggest that the concept of a *therapeutic continuum* is more useful than that of more rigidly bounded or discrete medical systems, between which individuals must choose." In sum, medical pluralism in Africa has been well documented and has informed this study. While there are broad parallels between the medical pluralism found in various African contexts and in Niger, unlike other studies I emphasize that while patients perceive a therapeutic continuum with fluid boundaries between sectors, healers do not see it this way. Healers think of the medical sectors as distinct and this is how they operate; that is, traditional healers dispense only traditional medicine and so on.

The key contribution of this book is that I take medical mistrust seriously. I do so first and foremost because Nigériens do. However, the mistrust–trust continuum is a dimension that has been overlooked or has not been a central part of the analysis in other studies. I argue that medical pluralism and medical mistrust are linked. Widespread medical mistrust has led to a situation wherein many Nigériens are not particularly invested in one particular sector and thus shop around for healing. While there are overlapping sectors from the perspective of patients, many Nigériens do not care which one works—they just want one to work. I also assert that it is important to take mistrust seriously because to some extent mistrust exists in all medical situations everywhere in the world given the inherent asymmetry in power between healers and patients. I emphasize that medical mistrust is not usually a pathology, but rather a pragmatic attitude and perspective for negotiating uncertainty. The generativity of the mistrust–trust model is that there is not a clear-cut distinction between the two modalities. They often coexist and it is precisely the ambiguity and uncertainty that opens a space where future therapies can be contemplated.

## Issa and His Father and Friends Experience
## Illness, Therapy, Recovery, and Death

Under a typical thatched roadside hangar and just across the street from an Islamic medicine shop in Abidjan, an old, poor neighborhood near the center of Niamey, a group of middle-aged and elderly men gather daily for hours for conversation. One afternoon in 2018 three men whom I have known for more than 20 years were enjoying each other's company: Aboubacar, Lamine, and Mamadou. Aboubacar is almost always there during daylight hours as he runs a typical small-scale business selling candy, cigarettes, peanuts, and condiments from atop a small table and his straw mat. He was having his head shaved with a straight-edge razor by Mohammadou, the best known *wanzami* (barber-surgeon) in the area. The primary daily work of *wanzamai* (plural of *wanzami*) is barbering. They also circumcise boys and perform bloodletting to remove "dead blood" from patients. About 65, Aboubacar left Gidan Kaza, his home village, 55 years ago. (Gidan Kaza is a village of roughly 1,000 residents situated 250 kilometers east of Niamey.)

Lamine, a 55-year-old tailor originally from the town of Filingué, likes to hang out here whenever he does not have a backlog of orders, which is typically several hours daily. He was receiving a manicure and pedicure. Many Nigérien men and women get manicures and pedicures about every two weeks, primarily because they are considered beneficial to health and only secondarily for cosmetic purposes. Thousands of specialists in Niamey trim nails, and most importantly, scape off layers of the nails with a scissors blade for 100 CFA (20 cents US). Mamadou, a 75-year-old man, also from Gidan Kaza, is a *d'ori*, a traditional bonesetter who also treats joint and muscle ailments with whispered incantations and spittle, was also there. In recent years, he has spent most of his time napping but will wake to treat a patient about every 30 minutes during the day. He never mentions a fee, but all his clients offer at least 200 CFA worth of coins for his therapy.

As I sat with my friends, 22-year-old Issa joined the older men. He is the son of Elhadji Anass—a prominent imam who operates a mosque and two Qur'anic schools across the street—and is studying veterinary science at Université Abdou Moumouni in Niamey. Tall, lean, and handsome, Issa wears elegant, flowing, white, embroidered Muslim robes on Fridays for the most important communal prayer of the week. On days when he does not have classes, he wears hip-hop clothing—baggy jeans, untied Timberland boots, a t-shirt, and a gold chain necklace. On days when he goes to classes, he wears formal trousers with a polo shirt or button-down shirt that are always freshly ironed. It is common for young men in Niamey to move between such different kinds of clothing. Issa's sartorial choices reflect that he is equally comfortable discussing Islam, science, music, football, and traditional Nigérien wrestling.

Issa respectfully greeted the men before taking a seat on a wooden bench. The older fellows had not seen Issa for a couple of days, and even though they had exchanged formulaic greetings about each other's health that had ended with "all is well" as is the norm, they inquired about the actual state of his health and where he had been. He had been suffering for three weeks with what seemed to be a bad cold. His father told him all along that Muslim prayer was the only path to recovery and that various medicines are pointless. Issa explained that he had visited a man recommended by one of his classmates in a village about 25 kilometers outside of Niamey. He explained that the man carefully examined the palm of his hand and then prescribed traditional plant medicine to treat his cold.

Virtually in unison, the old men exclaimed, "You saw a *boka*; this is *bokanci*!" *Boka* (sing.)—and *bokaye* (pl.)—is a Hausa term for "traditional doctor" or "wizard" who works with plants and spirits. *Bokanci* involves the work of the *bokaye*. Newman (2007, 22) also defines *boka* figuratively as "liar" and *bokanci* figuratively as "lying," revealing that mistrust of *bokaye* is embedded in the language. They laughed so hard that they had to pause for a few moments to catch their breath before they could ask their next question, "Did you pay him for this?" Issa responded, "Yes, 2,000 CFA for the diagnosis and medicine." Aboubacar, Lamine, and Mamadou laughed even harder—the kind of fall-off-one's-chair laughter that is so important to how Nigériens maintain their balance, dignity, and sanity despite dire poverty and troubled times. Issa attempted to defend his visit, explaining, "This is no different from the biomedical clinic where they use metal technology to look at your hands, in your mouth, eyes, and ears, and then diagnose and prescribe medicine. I had already tried the clinic—where I paid 4,000 CFA—and got no relief." He concluded, "I am finally much better, that traditional healer knows what he is doing." The older men took turns telling Issa that while a few *bokaye* have valid knowledge, most are charlatans who are also associated with *Bori*, the traditional Hausa religion. Issa again articulated a defense, "He was not a *boka*. There was no sacrifice and no spirit possession ceremony, so it was not *Bori*." Aboubacar was not convinced, "This is *bokanci*," and his friends agreed. Lamine added, "Next time, just buy some Kold Time from the mobile pharmaceutical vendors."

This encounter introduces many of the key dynamics involved in decision-making regarding navigating healing options in contemporary Niamey, namely, cultural identities and reputations, pragmatism, class, age, social networks, cost, and convenience. Issa's secure socioeconomic position meant that he had more healing options than many Nigériens, while his social network in which his religious father played a large role worked to limit the kinds of treatment he pursued. It also involved calculated role reversals. The three older men—who formed a "micro-community of mistrust" at least in the moment—almost certainly consulted with *bokaye* as youths in rural Niger, and probably still do so on occasion. Mamadou, the bonesetter, is a sort of specialist *boka* himself. All of them use traditional plant medicine purchased from street vendors. They expected that since Issa is a young, educated, middle-class son of an important Islamic teacher that he would know better than to consult a *boka*. Furthermore, despite their rural roots and lack of literacy, the older men desired to express their identities as modern, urban Muslim men.

I can only conjecture about the reasons Issa chose to tell his story. He had to know that due to his age, education in science, class, and status as the son of Islamic scholar that he was going to be picked on for sharing his story. Perhaps he wanted to show that he is more complex than they think—that he cannot be pigeonholed. Or maybe Issa just took pleasure at seeing his old friends laugh even if they thought it was at his expense. Lamine's logic drew from knowledge that a couple of days' worth of popular cold medicines can be purchased for 200 CFA (40 cents US) from *akwaku*, itinerant pharmaceutical vendors, who pass by about every 20 minutes throughout the day. Finally, Aboubacar, Lamine, and Mamadou questioned Issa's claim that he had been cured by a traditional healer and medicine. They suspected that he had actually been cured by his visit to the biomedical clinic and that the pharmaceutical drugs had taken time to achieve efficacy. Despite his public assertion, Issa may not be entirely confident about what made him feel better. After all, he chose to visit a clinic as his first course of therapy. Many Nigériens in Niamey use traditional, Islamic, and biomedical therapies simultaneously because they trust—or mistrust—each sector equally and because they want relief from suffering quickly and do not necessarily care what works so long as they feel better.

Death in Niger is shrouded in mystery. The consequences of illness can be severe, and people have to figure out how to make the best choices they can for themselves, but since illnesses are mysterious there often is not a clear path to the "right" kind of healing. When I returned to Niamey in 2019, much had changed since the previous year. On my first day I was eager to greet and hang out with the guys—Aboubacar, Lamine, Issa, Mamadou, and Elhadji Anass—I have known so long. Aboubacar and his table were not at his usual spot under the hangar, but soon Lamine showed up. He informed me that one morning a month before I arrived that Aboubacar had woken up mostly paralyzed from the waist down. Aboubacar's first choice of treatment was traditional medicine given to him by an old friend—a natural, plant-based salve stored in

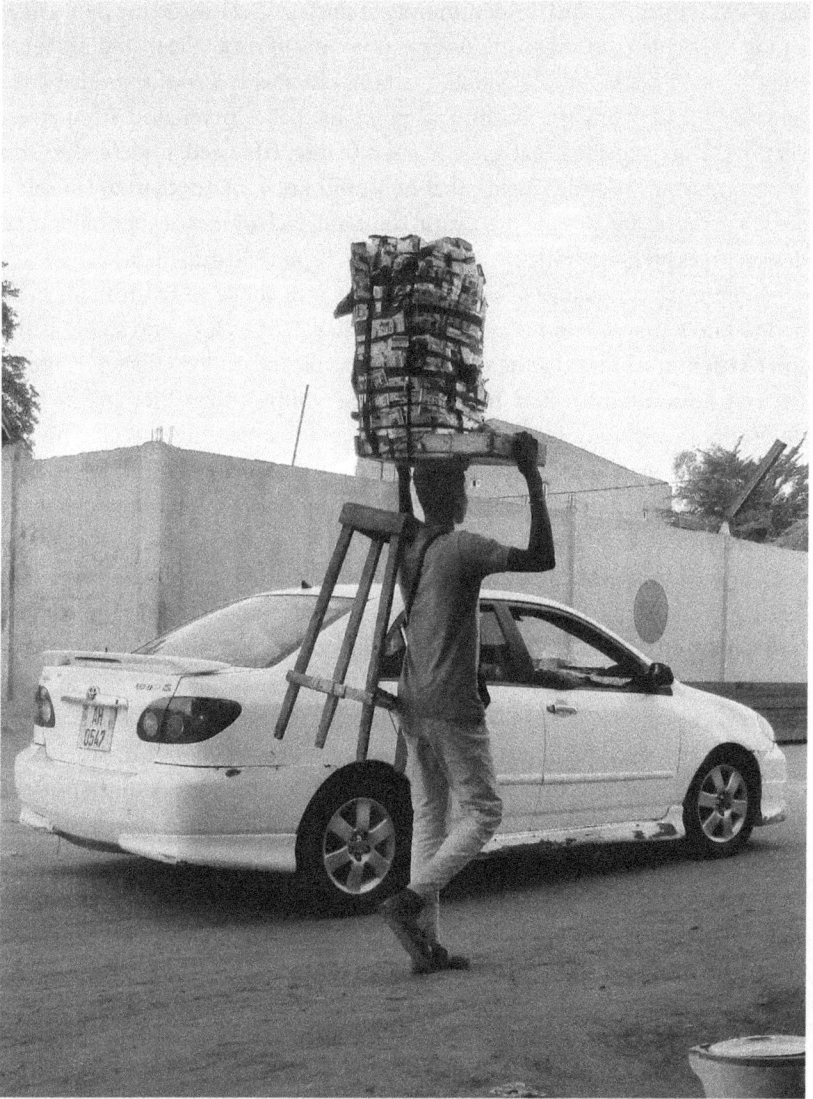

Figure 4.1. Itinerant pharmaceutical vendor with medicine tower on shoulder. Photo by author.

repurposed Nescafé coffee can. After that failed to provide any relief, he consulted with Mamadou, the bonesetter. Mamadou massaged Aboubacar's hips and thighs while whispering secret, magical words, but to no avail. Mamadou declared that the mysterious problem was beyond his powers to heal and recommended that Aboubacar visit a hospital. Lamine commented, "Even though he failed in this particular case, Mamadou proved that he is a healer of integrity who acknowledges his limitations and accepts that hospital medicine might work in some cases." Indeed, it is fairly common for healers in one medical sector to refer patients to another sector, though some healers insist that they can treat all conditions.

Aboubacar had never been to a hospital and expressed reluctance about going. He was nevertheless desperate enough to try anything, though I am not sure that he would have gone to the hospital if Mamadou had not recommended it. This illustrates the power healing networks have in people's decision-making in this mistrustful climate. One of his sons and a neighbor carried him into the hospital where he received an x-ray. Aboubacar reflected on the experience, "I regret going. I had no idea what to expect, and no one explained anything to me. They treated me without respect, like a boy. They acted like it [the partial paralysis] was my fault. It was awful lying on a cold metal table, and the smell—some strange chemical—made me ill." Medical doctors were unable to diagnose his ailment and sent him home with a pair of crutches. Aboubacar noted that this classic material item of primary hospital care was not useful, "I was too weak to use the crutches, and my son and his friend still had to carry me to a taxi." The next day, Lamine, Issa, Ali (also a migrant from Gidan Kaza), and I visited Aboubacar at his home in Dan Gao, a distant neighborhood, using a car that I had borrowed from a friend. We came with greetings and cash gifts. As traditional as Aboubacar is, there is nothing like the material culture of cash money to access food, medicine, and other essentials in a capitalist world. It is common in Niamey for friends to give each other money in these circumstances. Aboubacar was glad to see his friends and accepted our gifts, but as a proud man who had operated his little business almost every day for more than 40 years and had been strong and healthy all his life—except for losing most of his teeth over the years—he was embarrassed to accept help and by his pitiful predicament as he could only crawl with difficulty between his bed and a toilet. He died a week later.

Mamadou was not around the hangar in 2019 and I was told that he was too frail to travel from his neighborhood to the place where he worked. His decline had been gradual and was less surprising than Aboubacar's. By 2009 he could no longer safely ride his motorcycle to work but for five years after that he could still manage to hail taxis. For the next five years he had relied on his sons and friends to drive him to and from work. Lamine and I went to visit him at his home to greet him and see how he was doing. Mamadou explained, "I am so old that even the strongest traditional medicine cannot help me now. I have never been to a hospital, and I see no reason to start now. I am a traditional healer and that would be hypocrisy. I have lived a long life, I have helped people, and I do not want to be a burden to family." He died few days later.

Elhadji Anass, the father of Issa whose quest for healing was discussed at the beginning of this chapter, also died in 2019. I had known him since 1991 as the pillar of the Gidan Kaza community in Niamey, not only as an Islamic scholar but also as man who offered lodging to migrants, scholars, and travelers free of charge, regularly donated dozens of heads of livestock to poor neighbors during Muslim holidays, drilled a borehole to provide free water to neighbors and passersby, and so much more. For decades, he preached daily to small circles of colleagues and students and on Thursday evenings—the traditional time for public Islamic sermons in Niger—to audiences of 500 people using his powerful, distinctive, authoritative voice as well as clear, profound, and articulate use of Hausa and Arabic. His preaching over the years—among a wide range of topics—emphatically denounced traditional religious practice, such as *Bori*, involving spirit possession. In my estimation this emphasis may have been magnified by the reality that his home region and that of a core group of his congregants is one of the strongest bastions of *Bori* in Niger and the distinct possibility that his early years were spent in an animist family. Almost all of the Gidan Kaza diaspora community in Niamey strongly identify as a "pure" Muslims, including about two-thirds over the past two decades who have followed Elhadji Anass's lead toward austere Salafist practice with direct funding from an organization based in Saudi Arabia.

About a decade ago Elhadji Anass woke up unable to speak beyond a barely audible, raspy whisper. For a couple of years, he practiced what he preached, that Muslim prayer can cure all. He also regularly drank the common, traditional, Muslim-approved Nigérien treatment for colds, laryngitis, influenza, and, most recently, COVID-19—hot water with honey and lemon or lime juice and garlic. After getting no relief, he compromised and sought treatment in hospitals in Niamey, and then in hospitals in Morocco and Tunisia during the next few years. For a couple of weeks after he returned from his six-week visit for therapy in Tunisia he was able to speak at a normal conversational volume, but that did not last, and he was never again able to deliver sermons to large gatherings. Elhadji Anass shared with me that "I am highly skeptical of doctors, and the only reason that I tried them was because they were Muslims, even though most of them are not as serious about Islam as they should be. I hated the cold machines and needles. And where did that get me? Patience and faith are the only remedies for living in the world." He maintained his dignity and profound presence, shared that no clear diagnosis was ever made, and never revealed sadness about this.

My profiles of Issa, Aboubacar, Mamadou, and Elhadji Anass highlighting the onset of their health problems and their therapeutic itineraries reveal important recurring themes of the chapter. These include the prevalence of sudden crises; ways that maneuvering through medical systems is influenced by social identities, faith, and desperation; mistrust of healers and treatments; perceptions about the material culture of medicine; and a sense that spirits are always nearby.

Issa, Aboubacar, and Elhadji Anass experienced sudden and mysterious crises, though of vastly different degrees of severity. Issa evidently came down with a severe cold or influenza overnight and eventually recovered. Aboubacar's rapid decline took him from vitality to partial paralysis and death in a matter of weeks—an experience that, unfortunately, is typical in the lives of so many Nigériens. Elhadji Anass abruptly lost his powerful voice, and never recovered it, but was otherwise healthy during the last ten years of his life. Although it did not kill him, he lost a central element of his position and persona.

Their stories are not atypical. Life is hard in Niger. Virtually every Nigérien knows of a seemingly healthy family member or friend—from infants to elders—whose well-being abruptly declined, leading to long-term or permanent loss of some bodily function (ambulation, speech, hearing, continence), "madness," or death within hours or days. Most Nigériens never get a firm traditional or biomedical conclusion regarding their problem, or an autopsy, and thus family and friends are left to sort through a variety of explanatory narratives—natural or physical causes; attacks by witches, sorcerers, or angry spirits; and most prominently, that it was Allah's will, end of story. All this uncertainty and ambiguity contributes to mistrust.

The men navigated medical pluralism in diverse ways, and this was influenced by their social identities but not in simple or predictable ways. Issa is the most cosmopolitan and pragmatic man of the group. He casually and fluidly

moves between each health sector (traditional, religious, and scientific), seeing no contradictions in doing so, just as easily as he changes from his street
clothes and university clothes to his Muslim gowns. As a traditionalist and
devout Muslim, Aboubacar reluctantly turned to biomedical care as a last
resort. Mamadou elected to use only traditional medicine and justified this
as the proper thing to do as a traditional healer. Elhadji Anass, an Islamic
scholar and preacher, used Islamic prayer for two years to treat his ailment
before desperately compromising and visiting several hospitals, including
ones in Morocco and Tunisia. These examples show that navigating medical
pluralism in Niamey is a deeply personal process. Most Nigériens, even if they
are extremely devoted to one medical sector, seek healing in multiple sectors,
at least in extreme circumstances.

Issues of mistrust and trust are also evident in this case study. Aboubacar,
Lamine, and Mamadou mistrusted the healer that Issa consulted, because they
assumed that the healer works with spirits. Aboubacar, Mamadou, and Elhadji Anass deeply mistrust biomedicine. However, only Mamadou declined
to visit a hospital. Aboubacar and Elhadji Anass, like many people in this
impoverished nation, were desperate enough to overcome their medical mistrust to make sure that they tried their best to survive their illnesses. Mistrustful perceptions of the material culture of medicine are evident. Issa was
not impressed by the metal implements used to examine him, even though
he is being trained to use roughly similar ones in veterinary science. For him,
the biomedical diagnosis that he received resembled the diagnostic techniques
used by the traditional healer who did not use technologies, and he concluded
despite his background in science that the latter was superior. Aboubacar and
Elhadji Anass were extremely uncomfortable with the x-ray machines, cold
metal tables, and sharp needles that they encountered in hospitals. Mamadou
chose to avoid the material culture of medical technologies altogether. The
material dimensions of therapies play an important role in shaping Nigériens'
mistrust and trust of them.

Open expressions of mistrust and emotions are rarely evident in ceremonies surrounding death in Niger. Nigérien Muslims mark death with simple
rituals and with very little expression of emotion. To cry upon the death of a
loved one is considered as showing lack of faith in Allah's will. As soon as a person dies, the body is washed, dressed, and covered in a simple white shroud.
Family and friends who are nearby gather to pray. In rural Niger, the body is
carried on a bier to a cemetery and interred within hours of death with the

body and face of the deceased facing Mecca, the holiest city of Islam. In Niamey, people often take the deceased to a morgue to register the death before burial rather than going straight to a cemetery. Typically, no marker is used, though some families mark the site with a small flat plaque. The white shroud and simple grave marker, if any, symbolize people's humility and equality in the eyes of Allah. The deceased is commemorated in prayer on the third, seventh, and fortieth days after death. Streams of visitors arrive on those days, or whenever they can, to greet the family and share memories of the good qualities of the deceased. Some families host large receptions on these days. For example, Elhadji Anass' family rented plastic chairs and canvas tents that they erected in the wide road in front of his compound and mosque to accommodate the several hundred guests who attended the reception.

Despite the stoic, sincere, patient acceptance of death among most Nigériens as part of Allah's infallible plan, even the most faithful sometimes cannot avoid wondering if their kin, friend, or neighbor was victimized by a wizard or an angry spirit. A lingering sense that the spirits are never far away despite the austere "re-Islamization" (R. Idrissa 2017, Sounaye 2013) of Niger is demonstrated in the experiences of these men. I think Issa was open to the possibility that his cold was caused by a spirit, even though he denied it to his friends. Aboubacar and others wondered if the mysterious turn of events that impacted Aboubacar was due to a spirit attack or witchcraft despite Elhadji Anass' admonitions to ignore such "superstition." They quickly dropped the subject and stoically expressed faith in Allah's will after Aboubacar's death. Elhadji may have never considered that he was the victim of a spirit attack, but some of the people who knew him, and his plight, did. In private conversations in hushed voices before and after the reception, several of the men and women of the Gidan Kaza community in Niamey that I know well, and others that I spoke with during my visits to Gidan Kaza, shared with me their perspective that the spirits had found a perfect way of punishing him for his disrespect by depriving him of his voice. I am not aware of Mamadou or any of his friends attributing his death to spirits, and I think that there is an explanation. Unlike Issa, Aboubacar, and Elhadji Anass, Mamadou's ailments came on gradually. In Niger, the ever-present possibility of supernatural attacks makes diagnosing illnesses even more difficult since it adds another dimension, literally, that can cause people to fall ill. Furthermore, the spiritual element of illness contributes to a culture of mistrust as Nigériens sometimes suspect that they have been attacked by witches or sorcerers.

## Abdourahmane's Health Life History

Abdourahmane cut a classic Sahelien figure at 6' 9" tall and a lean 170 pounds with intensely black skin and high, angular cheekbones. He ambled elegantly and proudly and always wore what I call "West African business suits"— locally tailored suits made of imported black or gray polyester fabric—that were popular among civil servants in the 1970s and 1980s. Even though this style in now dated, he wore it well and it added to his aura of sophistication and intelligence. Abdourahmane was fluent in Hausa, Zarma, French, and English and spoke functional Fulfulde and Kanuri. He spent the second half of his life doing what most normal, underemployed men in Niamey do; he visited friends and family for daily stimulating, intelligent, and amusing conversation on topics ranging from the weather to world politics. Abdourahmane loved sharing jokes, proverbs, and laughter. Due to his life experience, he was comfortable with and showed respect for all people, regardless of wealth or education. I briefly introduced Abdourahmane as Mariama's husband at the opening of this book. Here I offer a synopsis of Abdourahmane's health life history with a focus on the ways that he has navigated physical and mental challenges as well as various forms of medical mistrust through his life course. My composite profile of Abdourahmane draws from our friendship of 31 years including a variety of encounters such as casual conversation, formal interviews, and traveling together to visit village market days in the general orbit of Niamey, as well as long journeys of 1,800 kilometers roundtrip to visit his parents and other family in a village near Zinder.

Abdourahmane led an unusual life in many ways. Thus, I do not claim that his life is typical of Nigériens. However, like so many Nigériens, he experienced a health crisis that radically altered his life trajectory. Abdourahmane was poisoned on the job by insecticides in 1986 when he was 31 years old. He lived another 36 years until he died in 2022, but he may never have fully recovered, faced a variety a variety of health problems, and never got his career back on track. My profile focuses on Abdourahmane's eclectic experiences navigating an enormous range of therapeutic options across all three primary medical sectors in Niamey. Like other Nigériens, he expresses contextual mistrust of healers and medicines, and yet due to his poverty and other factors he frequently lacked confidence in medical options that were accessible to him. Similar to the Nigerian man's quest for health discussed by Trovalla (2017, 147, original emphasis), Abdourahmane's "pursuit was *wishful doing*: actions made with an awareness of the uncertainty of outcomes and future perils but with a hope of bringing forth futures hoped for." Abourahmane was thus a "wishful doer" throughout the course of his life. He made decisions about his health options and continued to pursue a range of treatments despite lacking confidence in positive outcomes.

I have chosen to tell Abdourahmane's health life history in some detail, including some things that are not directly related to health, illness, and healing, because he was a person, not just a patient with illnesses. Abdourahmane was born in 1955 in Madoua, Niger, to a Fulani mother and a Kanuri father. Over the years, the family has come to consider themselves Hausa and they speak Hausa primarily among themselves. Moving between ethnic groups is fairly common and easy in Niger and plays and important role in cultural *brassage*. When he was born, his father accurately predicted that he would live until an old age but that he would face many health problems. Abdourahmane's mother had 12 children, while his father's two other wives gave birth to 10 children each. He fondly recalled that, "When we played pickup football games in our youth, we did not need to pick up anyone, it was me and my 10 brothers against any challengers." Abdourahmane's father was a civil servant and hence the family moved every few years while he was growing up, with stops in seven different cities across the 1,500-kilometer breadth of Niger from Niamey to N'Guigmi. Abdourahmane was recognized for excellence in mathematics, and when he graduated from high school, the government selected him for military service and a three-year, five-month training program in airplane engine mechanics in Algeria. After returning to Niger in 1981, Abdourahmane worked as a mechanic for the Nigérien Air Force for seven months. Then he was sent to the U.S. for two years for additional training provided by the U.S. Air Force before returning to work for three years in the Nigérien Air Force. This work included travel to many African countries, including state diplomatic missions. Once again, he was selected for more training, this time in France for eight months. Abdourahmane then returned to Niger for good in early 1986 to resume working for the Nigérien Air Force.

These were remarkable, formative, and memorable experiences for a young Nigérien man who grew up with kerosene lanterns, well water, and handmade mud brick homes in the Sahel. Abdourahmane greatly appreciated his training in Algeria, even though it was the first place that he experienced racism. He rapidly learned English in the U.S. where he met people from all five continents as part of his international cohort, lived through a snowy winter in Illinois, and rode horseback with cowboys on Texas prairies.

He was surprised that the lunchtime cafeteria at the school in France served wine and that French pilots and mechanics functioned effectively in the afternoons. In all these sojourns he focused on his studies, accumulated considerable mechanical knowledge, and also learned how to pilot small aircraft.

Abdourahmane's final stint in the Nigérien Air Force was incredibly frustrating. Even though he behaved humbly and as he put it "I always used my knowledge to work correctly," his workmates and most importantly his superior officers were jealous of and intimidated by the foreign training he had enjoyed and made his job intolerable. Instead of benefiting from his expertise, they ignored his input. As a result, he negotiated an honorable discharge from the military. In exchange for accepting foreign training Abdourahmane had sworn to serve for five years in the Nigérien military. He had fulfilled his commitment and though had envisioned himself spending his career in the Air Force and was disappointed, he figured that his skills would lead to other opportunities, and he was right. Abdourahmane shortly thereafter accepted an offer for a higher-paying position with the Ministry of Agriculture that was sponsored by the U.S. Agency for International Development (USAID) to maintain and fly crop dusters equipped with insecticides to combat locust invasions that periodically devastate agriculture in Niger. Meanwhile, with more flexible time, he met and married Fatima, a sophisticated, beautiful lycée (secondary school) graduate from northern Benin. She suffered a miscarriage and then gave birth to a sickly daughter. Despite this disappointment, Abdourahmane was in love and hoped to have many children with her. He was on a fast track to an upper-middle-class lifestyle with a cement villa, running water, and a car in the driveway.

Abdourahmane's career trajectory was abruptly disrupted in 1986 when he suffered severe chemical poisoning while operating a crop duster. He had not been provided with proper protective gear and nearly died. Abdourahmane spent three months receiving biomedical therapy in a hospital. He suffered respiratory difficulty, loss of appetite, and full body lethargy. Physicians advised him to stay longer but he did not think that his condition was improving and was terribly lonely in the hospital, so he traveled 900 kilometers east to convalesce at his parents' home for nine months, primarily with traditional medicines. In her work on medical pluralism, Stroeken (2017, 153) similarly found that among many Tanzanians, "When the hospital fails, hope is raised in traditional medicine." After a year of diverse traditional and biomedical treatment often taken simultaneously, a physician found him fit to return to work. When he asked for his job back, the Ministry of Agriculture claimed that they had found a replacement for him. Abdourahmane thinks that he was discriminated against due to not having connections with a new minister under a new president. While Abdourahmane was recovering Fatima, his wife, and the baby went to live with her mother. Once Abdourahmane returned to Niamey, they visited him several times. However, Fatima was frustrated by Abdourahmane's lack of income, and he felt shame in being unable to support his small family or to afford biomedical care for his unwell daughter. They decided to divorce and although in Islam men can claim custody of children, Abdourahmane agreed to grant custody of the child to Fatima. He figured that his daughter would be better off in his mother-in-law's compound with several women and children around to help Fatima than in his own empty compound. Abdourahmane occasionally wired them money when he could.

When I met Abdourahmane in 1991, he was still visiting the Ministry of Agriculture offices several times a week seeking work, but he was never rehired. Furthermore, he never found steady work again, only occasional short-term, low-paying jobs wiring houses for electricity, fixing automobiles, tutoring neighborhood children in mathematics, and selling blocks of ice from his two freezers to neighbors and fishmongers who work near his home. Life would have been even more difficult had Abdourahmane's father not allowed him to stay indefinitely in the modest mudbrick compound that he had purchased in the 1960s during one his posts in Niamey after he retired in 1985. Abdourahmane never dwelled on his misfortune and rarely spoke about it during the last 36 years of his life, at least when he was with me. However, when he was summarizing key experiences of his life with me in 2017, he reflected on a crucial decision, "My country is poor. They sent me to study abroad on the condition that I return to serve my country. Every once in I while, I ask myself, 'why did I come back?' I met many dishonest students who deserted and simply stayed in the U.S. and France. It is too late now. We are Muslims. You cannot change destiny. Besides, family is the most important thing to me, and I would miss my family if I stayed away for long." Abdourahmane's life was also shaped by the fact that he lived in Niger where there are no legal structures that would have enabled him to sue the state for damages.

Abdourahmane never seemed to be depressed despite the professional and personal setbacks that he endured. Instead, he maintained his dignity through his deep faith in Islam and meaningful connections with family and friends. Abdourahmane had to adapt to pauperization through stretching a thin and irregular budget, skipping meals during lean times, walking rather hiring taxis, and smoking cigarettes down to the filter. His life improved materially and personally when he met and married Mariama in 2000. For the next seven years, she earned most of the couple's income through her restaurant. However, when her sickle cell trait condition worsened in 2007 and compelled her to retire, they were back to square one. For a couple of years, they lived without electricity because they could not afford to pay the bills. Mariama suffered three miscarriages and the couple were never able to have children together. However, Mariama had three children from a previous marriage. In describing the course of his life, Abdourahmane emphasized that "No condition is permanent." This popular adage across many languages of West Africa, especially in Nigeria and Niger, comments on the shifting nature of the human condition. In Niger, poor or ill people use it to lift their spirits, whereas wealthy or healthy people use it remind themselves that success or happiness or health can be fleeting. This is also about finding balance, of not sinking too low or celebrating too much. Aside from fatigue, Abdourahmane did not seem to have any lingering side effects from the poisoning.

Islam was central to Abdourahmane's identity. He thought of his faith as a personal matter, rather than a public one. Abourahmane always performed the five daily prayers, but unlike many Nigérien men he usually preferred to pray alone or with a small group rather than in mosques. He fasted during Ramadan, respected Muslim dietary rules, and regularly gave alms to the poor despite his own poverty. Abdoudrahmane donned specifically Muslim men's attire—a flowing robe and skullcap—only twice a year for the two most important Islamic festivals, but he really disliked it. As he put, "I feel like I am wearing a tent instead of clothing." Furthermore, he had little interest in Islamic medicine, except for drinking vegetal chalk from Qur'anic slates to treat his itchy, bloodshot eyes every December through February when harmattan winds kick up Saharan dust. Abdourahmane's poverty prevented him from completing the pilgrimage to Mecca, but he was confident that "God will not punish me for this." He maintained good relations with his neighbors and a wide circle of friends, visited them when they were hospitalized and regularly attended their Muslim baby naming ceremonies, weddings, and funeral receptions. Abdourahmane acknowledged one "mistake," as he put it, in regard to his behavior, but he expressed no regrets. About six nights a year he enjoyed visiting bars to drink several bottles of beer. He reminded me many times over the years that Islam, at least in the way that it is interpreted in Niger, does not forbid cigarette smoking.

Abdourahmane smoked roughly one pack of cigarettes daily for the last 50 years of his life. Mariama hated it and constantly encouraged him to quit. This habit was undoubtedly detrimental to his physical health, but he truly enjoyed smoking Rothmans cigarettes and savored every drag.

Abdourahmane was quite energetic and seemingly healthy when we met even though he had already been smoking for 20 years and it was just five years after his poisoning. I was a marathon runner, but he had no difficulty keeping pace with me during our frequent long walks on searing hot days in Niger. However, Abdourahmane—like many or most Nigériens—suffered annual bouts of malaria during the rainy season that left him bedridden for two or three weeks at a time. He always used traditional herbal medicines to treat it. It was not that he trusted traditional medicine more than biomedicine for treating malaria, but it was what he could afford. In Niger financial circumstances dramatically shape people's choices, and traditional herbal medicines are usually the most affordable option. Abdourahmane trusted only traditional medicine, which he took about once a week, to treat heat–cold.

Despite his frequent use of traditional medicine, Abdourahmane in fact generally trusted biomedicine more than other forms of medicine. For example, unlike most Nigériens who clean their teeth with neem chewing sticks, Abdourahmane regularly brushed his teeth with a toothbrush and toothpaste. When he suffered cavities, he did not turn to traditional medicine or to traditional dentists who pull teeth from patients with pliers in open air markets as many Nigériens of his means do. Instead, through connections, he visited "night dentists." Night dentists are biomedically trained professionals who clandestinely re-open their offices late at night to treat patients for about one-half the cost of official daytime services. Keeping all his teeth into his 60s—which is unusual among poor Nigériens—was very important to Abdourahmane as a symbol of his association with modernity. He favored biomedicine due to his education and to positive experience receiving physical exams during his time in the military. Abdourahmane probably would have used biomedicine for everything—except heat–cold imbalance—if he could have afforded it. His example shows that even when a person prefers one medical sector, he or she may still draw from other sectors out of necessity.

Abdourahmane's health began to steadily deteriorate beginning in late 2018. He described his symptoms in 2019: "In the hot season, I can only walk about 100 meters before I tire and need to sit to catch my breath. In the cool season, I can walk 10 kilometers without any problem." He trusted biomedical professionals to diagnosis his problems even though he knew that he would not be able to afford pharmaceutical drugs. Abdourahmane was diagnosed with high blood pressure and an elevated heart rate. Following his physician's advice, Abdourahmane asked Mariama to use as little oil as possible in her cooking, and to stop including meat and high sodium Maggi sauce. He has also cut his pack-a-day smoking habit in half. He explained, "This has been hard. You know how we Nigériens love our meat, oil, and salt. And you know how much I enjoy my Rothmans cigarettes. Alas, I am now practically a vegetarian like you. I never thought I would see the day, but I want to live a long life like my parents." (Abdourahmane's father lived into his 90s and his mother is still living and reasonably healthy in her 90s.) Abdourahmane's physician also prescribed medication.[1]

However, Abdourahmane explained that he cannot afford to take it except during the hot season. During the other nine months of the year, he takes a concoction that he learned to make from an old friend consisting of equal parts of powdered (male) kola nuts and garlic that he adds to water and drinks: "It seems to work as well as the pills. Some of our traditional medicine really works. And it costs me next to nothing." Abdourahmane made practical choices about which medicines to take but favored biomedical treatment when he could afford it.

Abdourahmane's mental health changed considerably over the next two years in an alarming way. I did not notice this through our short phone conversations and texts during my two-year absence, perhaps because these primarily involved exchanges of standard greetings. I went to visit him at his home on my first day back in Niger in 2021—I could not go in 2020 due to the COVID-19 pandemic. He was not at home, but Mariama invited me in for tea. She informed me that Abdourahmane had been bedridden for four months and that he had started leaving home only in the previous week. She suggested that this was because he was happy about my impending visit. Abdourahmane returned and we exchanged warm greetings, before he lay down on a wooden table in his courtyard. This struck me as very odd because he always sat upright in chairs whenever we conversed, but I attributed this to his high blood pressure and the recent illness that Mariama mentioned.

I had no clue about the state of his mental health until the next day when he visited me at the home where I was staying. Following local custom, I offered him a glass of water at room temperature upon his arrival. Since it was the morning and I knew he liked coffee, I offered to make some. I returned from the kitchen with a cup of hot coffee and a bowl of sugar because I knew he took his coffee with a couple of lumps of sugar. Abdourahmane proceeded to add sugar to his glass of water. After he tasted it, he remarked, "Scott, this does not taste like coffee." I calmly responded, "That is because it is not coffee, you mistakenly put the sugar in your water." I was quite alarmed, but I tried not to show it. He then asked, "Are you sure that you did not try to trick me?" I replied, "No, it was a simple mistake that I sometimes make too, I will get you a fresh glass of water." I had no idea where our conversation would lead to from there. In fact, we really did not have a conversation. Rather, Abdourahmane launched into a three-hour monologue primarily on traditional divination and spiritual healing. I was tempted to interrupt him with questions but decided to let him tell his stories in his own way.

Abdourahmane began by informing me that he was very interested in the forthcoming two-week national conference on geomancy or divination. He explained that each of the eight regions of Niger would be represented, and that diviners from other Sahelian countries would also attend. Geomancers of different regions use different techniques and have different ways of interpreting them, though there is some overlap in methods. For example, he asserted that "Geomancy is international, everyone has a version," and mentioned interpreting cowrie shells "that are used by Black people everywhere," markings with sand on Nigérien calabash lids "as in Haitian Voudun," and water in calabashes. Abdourahmane indicated that diviners at the conference—assisted by interpreters—would investigate four subjects and compare their findings. These topics included the outcome of the rainy season that had just begun, projected agricultural yields at the end of the rainy season, the health of the population in the context of global COVID-19 pandemic, and a commercial forecast for the year. The meetings, according to Abdourahmane, were scheduled to take place at the Palais des Congrès—at the time, the largest conference venue in Niamey—and to be broadcast live on television as well as at multiple public video screens set up around Niamey. He added that diviners and the audience would be free to take breaks to pray, either as Muslims or Christians, and that during the conference Nigériens would be able to place international phone calls for the same cost as local calls so that people could inform distant family and friends of visions of the future divined at the gathering to guide their plans.

I found this story fascinating and surprising. Abdourahmane told it with such certainty that although I doubted this conference was real, I asked around and searched online for information about it just to be certain. There are no official national divination conferences that receive media coverage in Niger where geomancy is a private matter. I can recall only one occasion over three decades when Abdourahmane expressed interest in divination. On a visit to a rural market about 15 years ago we were both drawn to a vendor selling elaborate Islamic divinatory-protective posters featuring esoteric numerology, symbolism, and liturgy. However, because Abdourahmane regularly dismissed various non-Islamic traditional healers who work with spirits as charlatans, I was surprised by his apparently sudden interest in various forms of divination. Perhaps he sensed that his days were numbered and wanted to confirm this.

Abdourahmane, after a very brief pause, recounted in vivid detail a very personal story involving traditional healing. The events in the story never happened. I argue that the story is open to multiple interpretations and suggest that it features a montage of distorted memories from his experiences over decades. I also assert that this story is important to tell because it includes important issues about navigating medical pluralism and mistrust, details regarding traditional healing, the importance of therapy management groups, and "wishful healing." The story involves me and my family, and hence a little background context is important for trying to make sense of it. My first wife, Kiren Ghei, visited Niamey once in 1991 with our baby daughter, Jamila. Abdourahmane never met Kiren in person, but over the years was keen to briefly greet her during our telephone conversations. He came to know my second spouse, Sara Beth Keough, due to our mutual research trips to Niger from 2009 until 2018, all of which included our son, Reid, after he was born in 2010. Jamila came to visit Reid, Sara Beth, and me for three weeks during our yearlong stay in Niamey in 2016–2017.

Abdourahmane began by recalling that Jamila became "very ill" during her visit when she was 26 years old. (Indeed, shortly into her visit she experienced an upset stomach and stayed mostly in bed for two days, and I knew that Abdourahmane was aware of this at the time that it happened.) He explained that after "she did not get satisfaction" at a biomedical clinic, Mamoudou Djibo along with three other professors referred us to a traditional *duba* ("diviner-healer") in Gotheye, a village 80 kilometers northwest of Niamey on the banks of the Niger River. About 10 years earlier, I had visited Gotheye with Abdourahmane to enjoy the car ferry trip across the river and fresh fish. Abdourahmane explained that we traveled to visit the *duba* who was in his 70s and had begun practicing divination and healing at age of seven as part of the heritage of his family, like his father and grandfather before him. He described the layout of the healing hut as a circular structure about five meters in diameter with a soft sand floor and center pole to hold up its thatched roof, and quickly sketched a detailed map that included the positioning of two guards/assistants. Five calabashes with water—one each with egg, milk, honey, millet, and yams were spread out evenly around the perimeter of the healing space. Before proceeding, the *duba* confirmed that we eat each of these Nigérien foods. Then the healer asked Abdourahmane if he is left-handed or right-handed. He was instructed that left-handers should move clockwise around the hut, starting at the first "station"; that is, the egg and water, and to drink a mouthful from each station. Jamila repeated these steps at the five stations. After the first circuit, the *duba* added a powdered mixture to each station, and Abdourahmane and Jamila completed the circuit again. Meanwhile the *duba* performed several rounds of geomancy with sand markings while uttering phrases in Hausa and Zarma.

As Abdourahmane remembered it, the healing ritual took a dramatic turn when the *duba* hung a cloth in the hut, dividing it into two halves along a north–south axis. Abdourahmane, Sara Beth, and Jamila were instructed to enter behind the cloth while the two guards moved to the opposite side of the hut by the single doorway. Then, Jamila began "seriously vomiting with blood" and trembling in a trance. Sara Beth grabbed Abdourahmane and asked, "Is she going to die? Don't kill her!" and pleaded with the *duba* to stop. Then, Sara Beth began sweating profusely and drooling, but Abdourahmane by chance had tissues to help her. Abdourahmane intervened and announced to the *duba*: "I am Jamila's mother and her father—continue." Next, with a new mixture of powders, the *duba* burned some incense in a brazier. This also induced a trance in Sara Beth that included babbling in multiple languages and more drooling before she fell asleep and "We forgot about her." Abdourahmane explained that he was instructed to lift Jamila in his arms and embrace her because she is not too heavy while perfumes and peppers were added to the incense concoction. "Now is the real beginning—the foundation of his job," as he described it.

The seer put a large piece of fabric over Abdourahmane and Jamila and the incense mixture and then visited the five stations, uttering a magical language that was neither Hausa nor Zarma nor any intelligible Nigérien language. The *duba* asked Abdourahmane to rest for a few minutes because he was perspiring profusely under the cloth while tightly holding Jamila, or as Abdourahmane put it, "My pants were as wet with sweat as if I had pissed myself." The *duba* told him to be patient, that he and Jamila must suffer if they want satisfaction, before adding another incense mixture to the brazier. Abdourahmane recounted that the old diviner recognized that there is not only Allah, but many gods, "exactly like in India," and "spoke with them and shouted that Jamila's mother will be glad." Abdourahmane then explained to the *duba* that Jamila is the daughter of Kiren, himself, and me and that he and I are brothers. The *duba* said that Kiren was crying at home because of Jamila's illness before asking Abdourahmane if he trusts him. He responded affirmatively and they opened the fabric and found Jamila sleeping. Sara Beth was still sleeping until Abdourahmane shook her seriously to awake her. She was very weak and the *duba* brought another herbal powder mixture and instructed Abdourahmane to put some in her left ear, right ear, eyes, nose, and mouth in that order against her will before giving her mineral water from an unopened bottle. After Sara Beth stirred, the *duba* told Abdourahmane to tap her three times on the head. Then, he said to her: "Look at me seriously, I have something to tell you." Sara Beth asked, "What are you doing?" Abdourahmane responded, "The *duba* has a message for you." The *duba* then spoke to Sara Beth directly and said, "I can see you are suffering but everything is over now." Abdourahmane (emphasis added) happily informed Sara Beth that "You can keep *our* daughter; she is healthy now!" The *duba* then informed Sara Beth that "Jamila must eat, her belly is empty. You must force her to eat if necessary."

Abdourahmane, Sara Beth, and Jamila exited the healing hut to talk with Kiren who had spent a lot of money to fly to Niamey. In Abdourahmane's telling of the story, I had stayed outside of the spiritual venue for the duration of the healing process and that "It was an honor to render service because you are my brother." I asked him "Was it a spirit that attacked Jamila?" He replied, "It was not a spirit, only Allah." Finally, I asked him, "Did we pay the *duba*?" Abdourahmane responded, "The *duba* could see that we are all honest, and therefore he did not fix a price. I do not know if you paid him."

These two stories, especially the latter one, were told with remarkably vivid detail. Abdourahmane said he remembered the healing ceremony "as if it had happened yesterday." It was real to him. And they are coherent for the most part. Various forms of divination are practiced across Niger. Healing rites in Niger do involve the importance of cardinal directions, mystical powders and languages, incense, and trances. These stories raise many unanswerable questions. Most importantly, why did Abdourahmane, a proud Muslim, tell stories of traditional divination and healing? I knew that he regularly used various types of traditional medicine, but I also knew that in the past he detached plant medicines from connections with spirits, as many Nigérien Muslims do. Did his poisoning have anything to do with his condition? Why did Kiren move in and out of the story? Why were Kiren and I left outside of the healing hut? Why did Abdourahmane refer to me as his "brother" and to Jamila as "our daughter"? Were these kin-based associations and the successful healing of my daughter ways to show me that he deeply valued our friendship? Did he think of Jamila as his own daughter because he never really knew his own daughter and because each of his wives had miscarriages? Why did Abdourahmane put himself such a central role in Jamila's healing story, in a way emphasizing his own healing powers? These stories were simultaneously disconcerting and fascinating to me.

Several important themes of this chapter and book are evident in Abdourahmane's life history. Like many Nigériens, he navigates various healing sectors even though he generally prefers one, often due to financial constraints. Abdourahmane credited biomedicine for saving his life but also chose to convalesce in his parents' home with traditional therapies for his chemical poisoning against the advice of biomedical doctors. He mistrusted many healers and therefore relied on family and friends and other people that he considered trustworthy in his medical decision-making, as is typical among Nigériens. For example, through connections to an underground network within formal-sector biomedicine, he figured out how find "night dentists," accredited dentists who offer steep discounts after regular hours. A friend taught him traditional treatments for his hypertension. His telling of Jamila's healing involved a PhD and group of professors recommending a traditional healer.

Abdourahmane's rendering of Jamila's healing ritual is obviously idiosyncratic; however, I suggest that it might also represent how some Nigériens think traditional healing should work. His story may have been empowering for him as it reveals what it would be like to feel certainty in medical treatment. It may show what an ideal healing experience should look like: A Nigérien having power and control over a complex healing process even though an honest, lifelong traditional healer who did not ask for compensation is directing it. He helped guide the whole drama, from finding the famous healer through respected sources to showing great care for and commitment to Jamila's and Sara Beth's well-being in practical ways. His story also reaffirms the importance of family and friend connections in healing in Niger. Abdourahmane claimed to be a parent to my daughter and a brother to me. While this is not literally the case, it is another indication of the importance of people beyond healers in patients' therapeutic journeys. Finally, it is revealing that Jamila had no agency in the story. It is common for children and wives in Niger to have therapeutic decisions made for them by parents and husbands.

Before Abdourahmane left my home, he shared a very different kind of story. He recalled being invited to a diplomatic summit meeting held at the international airport in Niamey involving Russia's President Putin; U.S. Presidents Clinton, Bush, and Obama; and Niger's President Issoufou. Abdourahmane explained that when an uninvited man tried join the meeting that he grabbed the man's arm and threatened to kill him if he did not leave. He then demonstrated the action by grabbing his own arm with such force that I feared he would hurt himself. In my estimation, Abdourahmane was suffering from a form of dementia, but I am not that kind of doctor. I felt uncomfortable about sharing my concerns with Abdourahmane given the stigma that is often associated with "mental illness" in Niger. However, I felt that I needed to do something to help my old friend, so the following day I shared my concerns with Laouli, one of his brothers. Laouli thanked me, told me that he was not fully aware of his brother's mental state, and advised me to avoid Abdourahmane until he found some psychotherapy for him. Selfishly, perhaps, I asked Laouli not the mention to Abdourahmane that I had shared my concern with him because I did not want Abdourahmane to be angry with me.

Laouli informed me about a week later that he and another brother, Mohammadou, had taken Abdourahmane to see a biomedical psychiatrist. He explained that Abdourahmane angrily resisted this, arguing that he was perfectly fine, and that he probably would not have gone if Mohammadou had not also encouraged him to do so. In the next two weeks, Abdourahmane and I did not communicate except for one text message exchange that he initiated. He let me know that he was very angry with me, but he did not indicate the reason. I asked for an explanation but never received one. I figured that he deduced that I had said something to Lauoli, or that anger was a symptom of his dementia. Laouli never shared the specific diagnosis of Abdourahmane's condition, but he told me that he was prescribed medication. However, he explained that not only did Abdourahmane refuse to take the recommended dosages he also was taking various traditional medicines to treat his mental health that may have been negating the effects of the pharmaceutical drugs he was prescribed. I attempted several times to bid him farewell before I departed, but he ignored me. A few weeks later, Laouli emailed with news that

Abdourahmane was much better and that I should contact him. We spoke by telephone, and though he seemed fine, he also seemed to have no recollection of my recent visit. A couple of months later, Laouli contacted me to inform me that Abdourahmane had died. Through the wonders of WhatsApp, I was able to attend the funeral reception virtually and offer condolences to Mariama and his family.

## Conclusion

Sudden health crises are all too common in Niger. The famous heavyweight champion boxer Mike Tyson once said, "Everyone has a plan until they get punched in the mouth." Elhadji Anass was figuratively—and in a sense literally—punched in the mouth when he woke up one morning without his powerful voice. He had never planned to visit hospitals and did not for two years while he used traditional tea and Islamic medicine. He finally compromised and not only visited local hospitals but traveled to hospitals in Morocco and Tunisia. Aboubacar went to bed strong and fully ambulatory and was punched in the spine as it were when he woke up primarily paralyzed from the waist down. As a traditionalist and as a man with limited means, he first tried traditional medicines and massages, before desperately entering a hospital for the first time in his life. Abdourahmane was figuratively punched in the mouth when he was poisoned and woke up in a hospital ward. He acknowledged that his initial treatment probably saved his life, but, as he explained, "After the lonely weeks in hospital passed by with uncomfortable needles, tubes, and chemical medicines I was not making progress. So I decided to check myself out early and go to my parents' home and get natural traditional medicines from my family."

Medical mistrust is pervasive among Nigériens but it does not paralyze them or prevent them from making medical decisions. Nigérien patients do need full trust in healers, medicines, and their own therapy management groups to make choices and take risks to improve their health. Indeed, they usually do not fully trust their options. Most Nigériens navigate medical mistrust by zigzagging pragmatically among therapeutic options across all three major medical sectors in Niamey. Mamadou, the old traditional d'ori or bonesetter mentioned in the first vignette, is an outlier among the people profiled in this chapter in that he used only various forms of traditional medicine, but even he recognized that other healing modalities can be efficacious when he referred his suddenly nearly paralyzed friend, Aboubacar, to a hospital for treatment.

Navigating medical mistrust and pluralism, however, is not a random, willy-nilly, free-for-all among Nigériens. Drawing from my broader data as well as the case studies used in this chapter and others, several important patterns emerge that help describe medical decision-making, particularly decisions made "after the fact." Four key variables, in no particular order, that guide the ways Nigériens zigzag through the medical system stand out: (1) the type and severity of the illness; (2) the proximity of the patient–healer relationship in terms of physical, social, and power distances; (3) the perception or reality of "costs," including financial outlays for consultations, therapies, medicines, and travel expenses, as well as the potential loss of dignity or autonomy; and (4) social identities as well as personal preferences. This is only the proverbial tip of the iceberg because each of these variables are in continuous interaction with each other and any one or more of these broad variables may emerge as more crucial in a particular situation faced by a particular Nigérien. For example, Aboubacar, as a traditionalist, avoided biomedicine his entire life until he faced a sudden debilitating crisis that defied traditional therapies. Furthermore, when they can, Nigériens select healers with great care because of the cloud of widespread fear that some of them may use their knowledge and power to harm or kill them. Although my daughter's healing story narrated by Abdourahmane did not in actuality take place, the violence of the treatment he imagined or remembered illustrates this point. While the story ended well, it is not difficult to imagine that it could have ended disastrously. This includes traditional healers especially, but biomedical institutions, policies, and healers are also feared as having potential nefarious intent. Islamic healers are not thought by Nigériens in Niamey to have malicious aims, but many are denigrated and somewhat feared—especially the self-proclaimed Islamic pharmacists that have emerged in recent years selling new, unfamiliar products—due to a sense that they may lack precise knowledge about the dosages and the potentially lethal consequences of overdoses of their products.

It is not always easy to quickly identify types and severities of illnesses in Niger. Many Nigériens think that heat–cold illnesses and certain types of spirit attacks can only be balanced, or at least managed long-term, with traditional therapies and medicines. However, heat–cold imbalances lead to symptoms that are virtually indistinguishable other illnesses, which complicates diagnoses considerably. Constipation may be caused by heat–cold imbalance, a spirit attack, food cooked in rancid oil, or an infection. Issa was unsure of the causes of his ailment, so he sought diagnoses and medicines in all three medical sectors. Many patients, like Abdourahmane as well as his wife, Mariama, seek diagnoses in one medical sector but treat their illnesses with medicines from other sectors. Therapeutic choices change as symptoms progress or as some are perceived to have failed. I argue that the difficulties in diagnosing illnesses both increases the likelihood that people will seek various kinds of treatment and thus sustains three flourishing medical sectors while simultaneously contributing to medical mistrust more broadly.

Nigériens generally like convenience, which is why street healers across medical sectors are so popular. From sunrise to sunset and beyond, if one simply sits on any reasonably busy intersection in Niamey for an hour, one will see several mobile healers pass by on semi-regular routes. Medical shops and markets that include medicine are rarely more a few minutes away from Nigériens' homes in Niamey. Nigériens appreciate the street healers because there are, for all practical purposes, no restrictions on the types of medicines that they sell because existing laws are not enforced. For example, patients can avoid long, crowded waiting lines at hospitals where their illnesses—including ones that they may be embarrassed about—may become known to many strangers, by discreetly visiting *akwaku* who frequently pass by their homes or where they work or hang out. Some will make house calls for long-term, well-known clients. However, a long-term, chronic, and debilitating illness, such as Mariama's sickle cell trait discussed at the opening of the book, may lead patients to travel thousands of kilometers in their quests for healing, even entering conflict zones in the process.

In general, Nigérien patients have more trust in healers who are close to them in social and power attributes than healers who are distant socially, economically, and in the ways that they interact with patients. Nigériens, as highlighted earlier, prefer maximal awareness of options and autonomy in self-care guided by therapy management groups. Abdourahmane's story about Jamila's healing involved a therapy management group. He served as the entourage's leader after a group of professors recommended a renowned traditional healer. While Nigériens rely on healers in a relationship of "mistrustful dependency" (Pasquini 2023) they want to be treated with dignity and respect. They perceive formal-sector biomedical facilities as places where they risk losing their autonomy by being treated rudely and with reprimands and directives. As Abdourahmane put it, "The street pharmaceutical vendors, even on a day when I have a cough, simply sell me cigarettes without comment. In contrast the doctors I have visited in clinics tell me that I am a fool to waste my money on cigarettes and that I must stop smoking if I want to be healthy." Nigériens would use formal-sector biomedical treatment more if they could afford to do so and if they had more confidence that they would be treated with respect and offered multiple options.

The costs of medical treatment are a crucial variable and barrier in one of the world's poorest countries. Rough one-half of the poorest Nigériens in Niamey earn less than or have access to only 500 CFA daily (1 USD). Most of these Nigériens trapped in poverty simply afford cannot many basic formal-sector biomedicines, such as a standard course of amoxicillin that costs about 20,000 CFA. However, men and women in Niamey also weigh the costs of treatment that stretch beyond financial measurement. Even when Nigériens have some trust that biomedical specialists may help them and they can afford to visit them, they sometimes think that the potential "costs" of losing their dignity and autonomy—in the most extreme cases, forced hospitalization as was feared in the initial months of the COVID-19 pandemic—outweigh the potential therapeutic value.

Social identities play a crucial role in medical decision-making and in the forms of medicine that are most likely to be trusted and mistrusted among many Nigériens. As discussed earlier in the book, traditionalist, Muslim, and Francophone or modern are three broad social identity constructions in Niger. These forms of affiliation, however, are fluid, situational, and not mutually exclusive in the minds of many Nigériens, as Issa's alternating between Muslim and modern dress illustrates. For others, these are core identities that guide or direct their medical choices. Mamadou was a devoted traditionalist who only used traditional medicine. Elhadji Anass stuck with Islamic medicine for two years even though it failed to alleviate his problem, before reluctantly and with great mistrust visiting various hospitals. Even then he justified this decision in part by limiting his healing journey to hospitals in other Muslim countries. Issa and Abdourahmane, as educated Francophones, generally trust biomedicine more than medicine of other sectors, but both situationally trust some traditional and Islamic medicine. Other forms of identity can also significantly influence the ways Nigériens navigate medical mistrust, including ethnicity, gender, occupation, and age. Some Nigériens trust healers of their own ethnicity and mistrust those of other ethnicities. For complex reasons discussed earlier, men generally trust women healers more than male healers to treat "heat." Women primarily trust only other women for guidance and care related to fertility, pregnancy, childbirth, and postpartum concerns. Old people tend to be more mistrustful of biomedicine than young people, but this varies by education, class status, and particular illness. Nigériens zigzag through medical sectors in their quests for healing. However, their zigzagging is not random. Nigériens make carefully considered choices, although these may shift depending on the circumstances.

This chapter has focused on navigating medical mistrust in a fluid context of medical pluralism, but it is also important to note that many Nigériens have medical decisions made for them in hierarchically structured therapy management groups. Parents and grandparents make medical choices for treating their children and grandchildren. Some Nigérien husbands control the therapeutic trajectories of their wives. Elder family members, especially if they have lost their physical and financial independence, depend on family to care for them as assisted living facilities, nursing homes, and the like do not exist in Niger.

Almost all Nigériens zigzag through traditional, Islamic, and biomedical sectors and around healers and medicines they mistrust in their pursuit of healing and health. Their movements and decision-making are patterned, not random. In this chapter, I have shown that pragmatism and convenience, social proximity, financial and emotional costs, social identities, and other variables play out and influence each other in complex and unique ways in the tens of thousands medical decisions that are made daily by Nigériens in Niamey in a context of pervasive mistrust. However, when Nigériens face sudden health crises or a significant loss of income, their options are disrupted and they sometimes feel compelled to make radical decisions that they never contemplated making before, including accepting treatments that they deeply mistrust. In the following chapter, I will examine the different yet overlapping ways that Nigérien healers seek to overcome patients' mistrust.

# CHAPTER 5

## Overcoming Mistrust

On a hot morning in 2021, Alhassan wheeled his pushcart carrying 40 different pharmaceutical drugs up to a typical roadside coffee, tea, and baguette stand under the shade of a neem tree and adjacent to an Islamic medicine shop in the Yantala neighborhood of Niamey, just as he does two or three times daily. He is 50 years old and has worked as a mobile pharmaceutical vendor for 15 years, including the last eight years in Yantala. Alhassan did not need to announce himself as a pharmaceutical healer because he is familiar in the area and his profession is obvious. He greeted Ali, the coffee and tea vendor, and Mansour, one of Ali's regular customers whom he knows, with friendly words and handshakes and nodded to four other patrons whom he did not know.

Garba, who was drinking Lipton tea, asked the other men that knew Alhassan if he was trustworthy. They responded affirmatively. A couple of minutes later Garba approached Alhassan, to explain that he was feeling poorly with a fever, headache, and pain in his joints. Alhassan asked him how long he had been suffering from the symptoms and then touched his forehead. Alhassan declared that he had either influenza or malaria and concluded that it was probably the flu since it was the hot season. He then said, "I will sell you some flu medicine and I will be back here about the same time tomorrow. If it is the flu, then you should feel somewhat better tomorrow. If it is malaria, you will not feel better tomorrow, and I can sell you some malaria medications, which are more expensive." Alhassan returned late morning the next day at about the same time as the previous day. Garba explained that he felt somewhat better. Alhassan responded that he could see that Garba was not perspiring profusely as he had been the day before. He then sold him a few days' worth of flu medicine and recommended that he drink lots of water.

Like many street healers of Niamey, Alhassan deployed a range of strategies to earn Garba's trust. In an earlier interview, he explained to me, "I realize that people have options and that many older people do not trust me and my medicines. For example, we are standing next to an Islamic pharmacy and under a neem tree that has many medicinal uses. I make myself available, I treat people respectfully, and I am always well stocked with good medicines." Alhassan is a relatively successful itinerant pharmaceutical healer in part because he has some medical knowledge. For example, his use of one medicine to confirm his diagnosis is not only a common practice among street healers across medical sectors but is also used by biomedical physicians. More importantly, I argue, "soft skills" have contributed to Alhassan's success. He is a familiar presence who is integrated in the community life of the neighborhood. This allowed Garba to ask Ali and Mansour for an assessment of Alhassan's character before he approached him. Garba was thus influenced by this impromptu therapy management group. Alhassan showed humility by declaring that he was not absolutely certain of the nature of Garba's illness. This strategy is common, though it is equally common for street healers of Niamey to express no doubt or ambiguity to project authority. Finally, by offering a less expensive medicine for a less serious illness rather than generating more short-term profit by recommending more expensive medicine for malaria, Alhassan may have gained a long-term patient. Alhassan also likely solidified his reputation among all the men at the coffee stand because they witnessed and overheard his interactions with Garba.

I have argued throughout this book that we must take medical mistrust seriously, in nuanced ways and in shifting contexts. I have emphasized the widespread mistrust of healers and medicines across all medical sectors of Niamey to this point. I turn my attention now to the strategies used by street healers to overcome the mistrust of Nigériens. In contrast with well documented examples of African patients' mistrust of biomedical facilities and crisis-framed public health policies, the strategies used by informal- and formal-sector healers to earn the trust of patients has been noticeably understudied. I argue that a holistic understanding of medical mistrust requires consideration of both sides of the patient–healer relationship (cf. Pasquini 2023). Traditional, Islamic, and biomedical street healers of Niamey compete against one another and with formal-sector biomedicine in a pluralistic medical context in which patients see a therapeutic continuum and "a sufferer must shop their sickness around" (Roberts 2021, 11), even while healers of each sector regard their practices as distinct from other sectors.

Medical mistrust and medical pluralism in Niamey are linked in a complex and seemingly paradoxical relationship. The historical, religious, social, and economic complexity of Nigérien cultures simultaneously makes it challenging for medical sectors to win patients' trust while also leaving room for diverse sectors to flourish. Indeed, mistrust can be a practical way of engaging with uncertainty. In some ways, then, mistrust inadvertently helps to maintain multiple medical approaches since mistrust of one or more sectors boosts confidence in a particular sector (even though Nigériens may not fully trust these healers). That is, I argue that *mistrust is productive*, even as it is frustrating and sometimes constrains people's healing practices and ability to make a living as healers. However, the impact of widespread mistrust is that it helps provide people with many options for healing, helps provide jobs for healers, and helps maintain a variety of cultural traditions just as it also helps people respond to uncertainty and rapid cultural change.

There is no one-size-fits-all way for Nigérien healers to overcome their patients' mistrust. Thus, I argue that it is important to pay attention to the *nuances and variations* within each sector and between sectors in terms of how different practitioners must do different kinds of work with different kinds of patients to gain trust. What works in one sector may not work at all in other sectors. In a series of groundbreaking, collaborative studies, medical anthropologists Anita Hardon, Sjaak van der Geest, and Susan Reynolds Whyte emphasized the importance of studying the material culture and "social lives of medicines."[1] This vein of research has faded in recent years, but I argue that it can yield important insights on medical mistrust, and I suggest that scholars should pay attention to *material culture* as they consider questions of mistrust elsewhere. I assert that creative manipulations of the material culture of medicines, medical packaging, and medical displays are important ways through which Nigérien healers of all sectors deal with mistrust. Healers of different sectors do so in very different as well as overlapping ways and in response to other sectors.

Traditional, Islamic, and biomedical healers who work on the streets of Niamey must exert enormous energy to earn potential patients' trust because Nigériens are often deeply mistrustful of all three sectors. Healers—especially traditional healers and informal-sector pharmaceutical healers—understand they are often mistrusted and seen as frauds, and they are also aware that they face competition within their own sectors and with rival sectors. They can sense glances of disapproval on the street; they notice the skepticism of some of their clients; and they realize their reputations are always at stake as they sell medicines that might not work or possibly worsen the health of their patients. Healers also know that they are mistrusted for different reasons. Healers simultaneously know that they have power in asymmetrical healer–patient relationships; that is, they are cognizant that Nigériens rely on them in relationships of "mistrustful dependency" (Pasquini 2023) and that a vast majority of Nigériens simply cannot afford formal-sector biomedical care even if they trust it enough want it. I will begin with a brief overview of core reasons that lead to mistrust of healers and healers' awareness of these reasons. Then I will analyze the strategies used by healers of each sector to overcome or at least alleviate the mistrust of Nigériens, including ideological appeals, self-presentation, styles of interaction with patients, and the creative manipulation of material culture.

Traditional healers know that some Nigériens fear that they can use their esoteric knowledge and power to harm people. They are aware that many Nigériens think they work with spirits and that this is increasingly considered evil and dangerous in Niamey given the rise in prominence of Salafist Islam. Even though most healers are not involved in *Bori* and other traditional religions that involve placating and negotiating with spirits some are, and this is enough to generate suspicion regarding all traditional healers in the minds of some Nigeriens. In addition, they know that they are stereotyped by some Nigériens as selling illicit drugs, such as marijuana, opiates, and cocaine, to supplement their incomes. Nigériens, through their understanding of Islam as well as local sensibilities, tend to regard the sale and use of these illegal drugs—even marijuana—as sinful and think that they lead users to depravity and madness. Though Nigériens vary widely in their perspectives on spirits, the former view of traditional healers is largely accurate in that many learn healing knowledge from spirits. The latter view is inaccurate because traditional healers do not sell illicit drugs.[2]

The media in Niamey occasionally offers reports of healers or sorcerers who kill children for their internal organs, especially hearts, or exhume graves in search of body parts to be used as ingredients in powerful magical potions. These stories or rumors periodically circulate in the city and heighten Nigériens' mistrust of these healers. Finally, two traditional healers in my sample identified charlatans in the profession as a problem that tarnishes their image. A 55-year-old Hausa traditional healer explained that "There are many amateurs in this business who lie and spoil our reputation."

Regardless of the veracity of these stereotypes, traditional healers must navigate these multiple sources of mistrust.

Mistrust of Islamic healers is correlated with their ages and the products they sell. Elderly Islamic healers who use longstanding, local Islamic medicines that are dispensed in simple packaging such as newspaper or coffee tins are usually trusted. In contrast, younger Islamic healers, who are calling themselves "Islamic pharmacists" and introducing new, imported medicines dispensed in industrial manufactured packaging, are viewed with skepticism by many Nigériens who worry that they care more about profits than healing.

Itinerant pharmaceutical healers are keenly aware of the long history of deep mistrust of biomedicine among Nigériens. Indeed, most of them have never or have only seldomly visited formal-sector hospitals, clinics, or pharmacies either because they do not trust them or because they cannot afford it. They know that many Nigériens regard them as charlatans who have no idea what they are doing and as entrepreneurs rather than "real" healers. Furthermore, many of them—especially those who are new to the profession—know that there is some truth to this. Many learn their genre of expertise on the fly by relying on general, public knowledge of pharmaceuticals. As discussed in earlier chapters, *akwaku* offer diagnoses and treatment suggestions, but most of their work involves simply selling whatever clients request. They also live with a low-level but persistent fear that their goods could be confiscated, and they could be shut down altogether at any time if the state ever chose to enforce existing law that restricts the sale of pharmaceutical drugs to licensed pharmacists (République du Niger 1997).

Table 5.1 shows demographic data on street healers of the three major medical sectors, revealing some important differences across sectors as well as some key similarities. Healers of each sector regard their practices as distinct. They do not mix medicines. Traditional healers sell only traditional medicine, Islamic healers use only Islamic medicines, and itinerant pharmaceutical healers dispense only pharmaceutical drugs. None of the healers interviewed put any limitations on who they are willing to treat, including Islamic healers who offer their services to "pagans" and Christians.

Gender is significant cause of difference and mistrust that must be overcome in healer–patient relationships. Almost all generalist healers across all three medical sectors who work in public spaces of Niamey are men, including 121 of 124 healers in my interview sample. Nevertheless, traditional healers of Niamey find ways to attract women as patients. Nigérien women consume the traditional and pharmaceutical medicines peddled in

Table 5.1. Demographic Profile of Street Healers of Niamey

| | | *Traditional Healers* | *Islamic Healers* | *Biomedical Healers* |
|---|---|---|---|---|
| Ideology | | local heritage | Islamic | modernity, science, practicality |
| Clothing | | Muslim more than Western | Muslim | Western more than Muslim |
| Gender | | 40 men<br>2 women | 21 men<br>1 woman | 60 men |
| Ethnicity | | 15 Hausa<br>13 Zarma<br>12 Fulani<br>2 Tuareg | 12 Hausa<br>8 Zarma<br>2 Fulani | 3 Hausa<br>37 Zarma<br>10 Fulani<br>7 Tuareg<br>2 Songhay<br>1 Zarma/Fulani |
| Age | average<br>range | 55.1 yrs<br>32–84 yrs | 42.3 yrs<br>28–64 yrs | 29.4 yrs<br>19–58 yrs |
| Prof<br>Exp | average<br>range | 22.6 yrs<br>14–69 yrs | 12.5 yrs<br>3–23 yrs | 5.9 yrs<br>months—25 yrs |
| Material<br>Culture | mobile | 11 mobile with sack<br>8 mobile with pushcart<br>3 mobile with car | 2 mobile with pushcart | 34 mobile with tower<br>12 mobile with pushcart |
| | stationary | 14 mat on ground, fixed spot<br>6 market stall | 13 boutique at mosque<br>7 stand-alone boutique | 10 fixed pushcart or table<br>4 small boutique |
| Neighborhoods | | 12 Boukoki<br>7 Gamkalle<br>7 Karadje<br>4 Katako<br>4 Dar es Salam<br>3 Aéroport<br>3 Saga<br>2 Wadata | 6 Abidjan<br>4 Yantala<br>4 Saga<br>3 Zongo<br>3 Nouveau Marché<br>2 Grand Marché | 15 Kirkisseye<br>11 Pays Bas<br>9 Banga Bana<br>5 Saga<br>5 Lambordé<br>3 Abidjan<br>3 Zongo<br>2 Nialga<br>2 Gawaye |

Table by Warren K. Fincher.

the street healing cultures of Niamey at roughly the same rates that men do. They account for almost 40 percent of the customers who directly purchase medicines in the traditional and biomedical sectors. Women of Niger are less interested than men in Islamic medicine as offered in public places, but they still make up about 20 percent of all customers. In addition, many Nigérien husbands purchase medicines for their wives. This is not the only example of cross-gendered healer–patient relationships in Niamey. Recall that women healers dominate the public market for treating illnesses associated with heat–cold imbalance, as I highlighted in Chapter 2. Despite pervasive gender inequality and segregation, Nigérien men and women recognize their mutual interdependence.

### Traditional Healers in Niamey Overcoming Mistrust

Traditional healers use appeals to Nigérien pride in local, cultural heritage to attract patients as they offer diagnoses, recommend therapies, and sell medicines on the streets of Niamey. They also draw on local understandings that local illnesses require traditional medicines to manage or cure. This includes illnesses associated with heat–cold imbalance as well as illnesses caused by spirits, sorcery, and witchcraft. Traditional healers consistently advertise that their medicines are natural, plant-based, and *bio* (organic) as they have always been. They do so either by word of mouth with their customers or through the labeling they put on medical packaging or on their banners. Not only do they emphasize the value of natural healing through plant medicines but they also warn patients about the dangers of pharmaceutical drugs made with unknown chemicals in faraway places that are designed for non-Nigériens. Most healers most of the time announce the types of ailments that they treat, not the specific plant medicines and recipes that they use. They will, however, when questioned, discuss with clients some of the specific plants that they use, especially if they are commonly known plants.

Traditional healers emphasize their long-term or lifelong commitment, that their healing knowledge was acquired by "inheritance" and training from either the fathers and grandfathers or mothers and grandmothers or both. By "inheritance" they mean that healing ability is passed through blood and that they were born with it. However, inheritance alone is insufficient, as would-be traditional healers study under their parents for at least 15 to 20 years before they are ready to practice on their own. Thirty-one of the

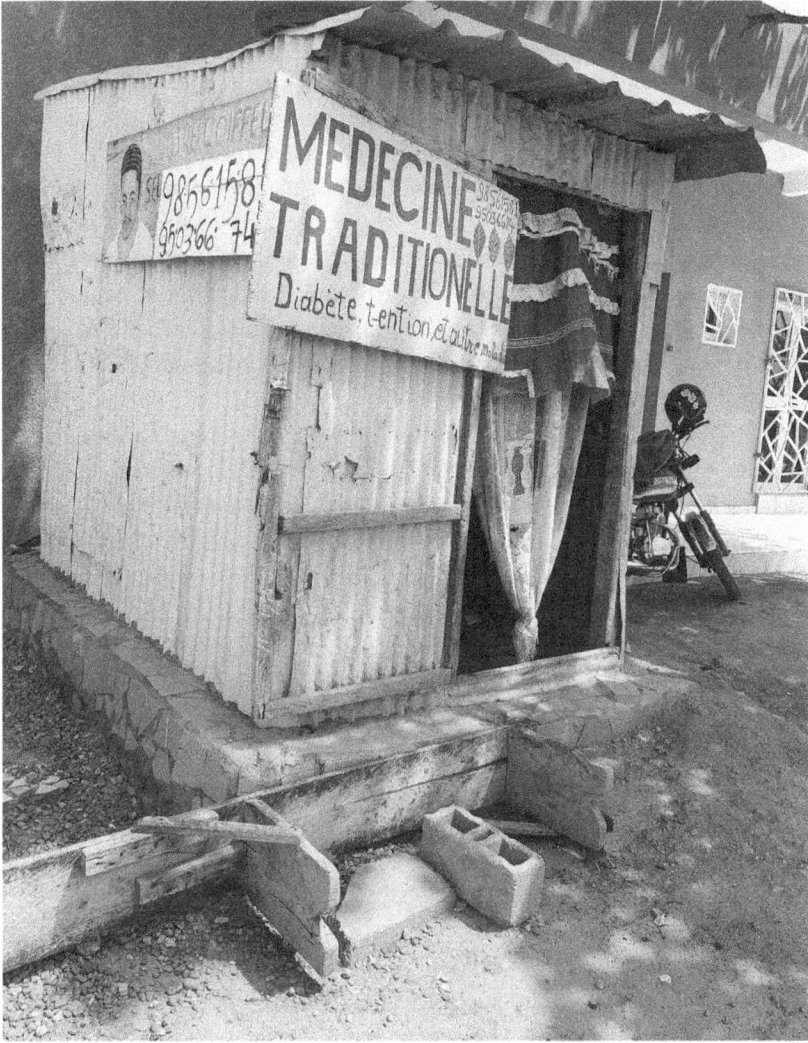

Figure 5.1. Traditional medicine shop. Photo by author.

42 traditional healers reported that they inherited this trade, including 21 who indicated that they inherited the occupation from their fathers, and 10 who indicated that they inherited the occupation from both their fathers and their mothers. Inheritance is not the only way to become a traditional healer. Those who did not inherit this trade could not just jump into it; rather, they

had to serve apprenticeships for years with established healers before they worked independently.[3] Most traditional healers explained that they have been working as healers for their entire lives beginning as children. They indicated that they share this commitment with their patients, not just with me. In a representative comment, one healer stated matter-of-factly, "It was the only occupation my family considered for me." This extensive training and knowledge sets them apart from most itinerant pharmaceutical healers and some Islamic healers, and thus is something traditional healers stress when trying to gain patients' trust. Furthermore, they are on average considerably older than Islamic healers (by 13 years) and biomedical healers (by 25 years) and realize that in most contexts Nigériens trust older people more than they trust younger people.

These healers did not merely adopt their work because it was expected of them; most take great pride in their work and express confidence in their abilities. Twenty of the 42 traditional healers interviewed mentioned that their work is a calling that allows them to earn a living to support their families. One-third of traditional healers in the sample—14 of 42—emphasized the role that they play in helping people. Many offered similar comments that reveal their sincerity about their healing power, such as: "I help the population to be in good health." "I help poor people regain health." "I heal those suffering from sickness." "I render a valuable service." "It is a dignified way of meeting people's needs." Others mentioned that they enjoy continuously building their knowledge and that their work allows them to get to know many people. Emphasizing this calling's noble purpose helps them to gain the trust of patients.

Traditional healers work to disassociate themselves in the minds of their clients from connections with spirits. This is especially true for older healers, who are aware that as they age, they risk generating more fear from people that they have honed their powers and may use them to harm or kill people. They typically wear clothing that marks them as Muslim and perform their daily prayers alongside neighbors, passersby, and clients in mosques and markets and on the street, signaling that they are Muslim and not affiliated with spirit possession traditions. One healer in the study acknowledged participation in *Bori* when he visits his home village but maintains a Muslim social persona in Niamey where he works and lives. Many Nigériens compartmentalize their religious lives in this way (Youngstedt 2013). Healers do so because of the generally negative reputation of local traditional religions in Niamey.

A variety of strategies are deployed by traditional healers to generate trust in their integrity and knowledge, and in the efficacy of their medicines.

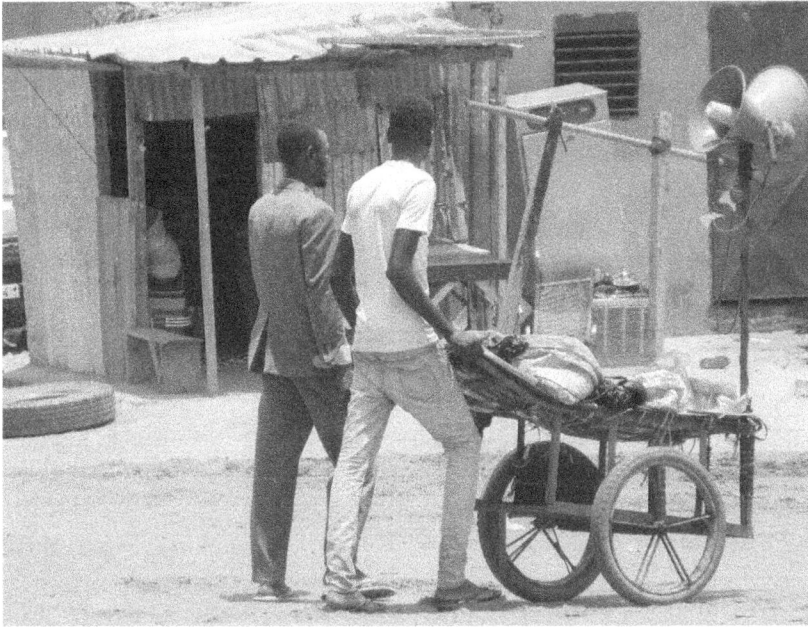

Figure 5.2. Traditional healers with plant medicines on pushcart. Photo by author.

They offer *convenient access* to traditional medicines as they ply regular daily routes in their neighborhoods and thus have some regular patients. Everyone in Niamey lives within a 20-minute walk of markets where traditional healers congregate, and mobile healers pass by on every reasonably busy street every 20 minutes. They can easily be found since they typically work about eight hours a day, seven days a week. The job is physically challenging for those on foot with sacks or using pushcarts. This marks them as regular people who are willing to spend hours a day in the hot sun of Niamey, as people of the same social milieu as their patients.

Marketing strategies are also important ways of making potential clients aware of their medicines and correlated with the degree to which healers are mobile. Some traditional healers quietly sit at fixed locations and wait for customers while displaying their goods in markets. Healers on foot make simple declarations that they are selling traditional medicine as they travel along the streets of Niamey. Those with pushcarts typically use megaphones to announce the main illnesses that they treat. Healers with cars use megaphones or loudspeakers to advertise their products, and when they park, they often set up 5- by 10-meter banners that list the conditions that they treat. Some traditional healers also make house calls and extend credit to long-time clients.

These healers *interact with patients respectfully*, observing local rules of etiquette and greetings in patients' languages and they are willing to be discreet when clients demand it. For example, traditional healers walk around the block to complete transactions with patients who do not want family and friends watching them for various reasons. This is particularly important for garnering women patients who strongly prefer privacy. Clients are slightly more likely to visit healers of their own ethnicity than of other ethnicities, but ethnicity is only one variable in their decision-making, and in many cases not the most important one. Convenience, cost, and the reputation of the healer are also crucial variables, and the latter can trump other considerations. (Recall Mariama's quest for healing that opened the book. She is a Hausa woman who traveled the length of Niger to visit a famous traditional male Kanuri healer.)

Traditional healers provide *affordable primary health care* to Nigériens in Niamey. Their therapies and medicines in most cases are far less expensive than the Islamic medicines or biomedical pharmaceuticals offered by their street rivals—and exponentially less expensive than formal-sector hospitals, clinics, and pharmacies for treatment of the same illnesses. That is, traditional medicine to treat malaria costs roughly 1,000 CFA; Islamic medicine to treat malaria runs about 1,500 CFA; street pharmaceuticals for malaria treatment sell for about 2,000 CFA; and formal-sector biomedical drugs to treat malaria cost about 8,000 CFA.[4] None of the healers in the sample charge consultation fees for their diagnoses—which I argue is another strategy for overcoming patients' mistrust. However, clients are expected to buy at least some medicine, especially if the healer has spent a lot of time with them. Many clients—probably a majority—do not seek diagnoses but are simply looking to buy specific medicines. Healers typically name more or less set prices for their medicines, but not always. Some healers, especially older ones, do not name prices, especially when they are dealing with regular customers. Instead, they ask clients to pay what they can or what they think it is worth to them. One 60-year-old Zarma healer explained, "My strategy of not asking for a certain amount of money adds to my credibility. Plus, there is a bonus: Clients often give me more when I do not name a price than when I do!"

Nigérien traditional healers recognize that they compete for patients with Islamic healers and especially with healers who sell pharmaceutical drugs, given their rapid rise in popularity over last 25 years. Many traditional healers—and Nigériens in general—have come to respect the power of bio-medicine to diagnose and treat illnesses of natural origins, especially through technologies and procedures such as x-rays and surgery. Many healers have learned and now use French biomedical terminology for anatomy and dis-eases, which also helps them assert their legitimacy and authority. Patients who get x-rays in clinics typically are sent home with large copies of them. These then circulate and are studied by many people in Niamey, including traditional healers.

Some traditional healers emphasize their knowledge and power as a means of alleviating patients' mistrust, whereas others humbly acknowledge their limi-tations to establish legitimacy with patients. This pride–humility continuum plays out in relation to traditional healers' interactions with biomedicine. Twenty-two traditional healers in my sample of 42 do not interface with bio-medicine and do not refer patients to hospitals. Seven emphatically empha-sized that this is not necessary. As one 50-year-old Hausa healer put it, "I do not send clients to the hospital; I have medicines to treat all conditions." In contrast, 20 healers explained that they have professional connections with biomedical practitioners. They refer patients to hospitals for a variety of conditions, including general checkups (four mentions), "complicated prob-lems" (three), eye problems (three), paralysis (two), edema (two), intestinal problems (two), migraine, cough, cyst, abscess, AIDS, vomiting, complicated kidney problems, and complicated hypertension. Long-time healer Rabiou described his strategy for earning the confidence of patients: "I can treat many illnesses with my plant medicines, but not all of them. Healers who claim they can cure everything are not honest and endanger the lives of their patients. My patients appreciate my honesty." He added that he recommends that some of his patients visit hospitals and that this helps build confidence in his integrity.

Eleven of the traditional 42 healers reported that they receive clients that hospital workers sent to them to treat a range of problems, including jaundice (four mentions), bad spirits and djinn (two), edema (two), goiter, joint pain, diarrhea, and dental problems. A traditional healer with 30 years of experience proudly explained, "Even modern doctors recognize that I have medicines that work. Because they send their patients to me, the patients have trust that I can help them." Several traditional healers mentioned exchanging health and healing information with biomedical physicians, and one regularly works the public health agents. Two mentioned that biomedical doctors request certain traditional medical potions from them for their own use.

Traditional healers of Niger also seek to overcome patients' mistrust and promote their credibility through "professionalization" (Last and Chavunduka 1986). A small group of traditional healers founded the Association des Tradi-Praticiens du Niger (ATPN) and registered it with the state in 1995 as an official NGO. This was about the time that pharmaceutical drugs first appeared for sale on the streets of Niamey. Traditional healers are the only healers in the informal sector who have established a formal association, and traditional healing is the only occupation in the informal sector with an institutionalized organization. I argue that traditional healers founded ATPN because they are acutely aware that they are widely mistrusted by Nigériens even though they take their knowledge and therapeutic role very seriously. Furthermore, the emergence of ATPN is an important development that illustrates many of the themes that I have explored in this book and in this chapter;[5] namely, interactions between traditional and modern medicine, traditional healers change and adapt transethnic traditional healing in Niamey, and healers' interest in solidifying their public credibility. ATPN now has more than 3,000 members—about 80 percent are men—across Niger. Its Board of Directors reside in Niamey where they rent a small office and includes a president and six officers. They range in age from about 50 to about 75 years old. Their official membership book includes a photograph, name, place of residence, and medical specialties, if any, of each member. ATPN is explicitly apolitical. Anyone can join for a fee of 1,000 CFA, though wealthier people are expected to give more. This organization seeks to defend and promote traditional healing throughout Niger, despite its shoestring budget. Directors emphasized that the bush—the source of most traditional medicines—is being depleted by urban growth, the expansion of farms, and climate change. They have established a few small botanical gardens to preserve particularly useful plants and access to them and hope to expand these operations.

The president of ATPN argues that members of the association are perfecting traditional medicine by combining the knowledge and best practices of healers across Niger's cultural groups. Indeed, the president is a Hausa man, and the board consists of two Hausa men, a Zarma man and a Zarma woman, a Tuareg man, and a Fulani man. Similarly, members come from all Nigérien ethnic groups, live throughout Niger, and are primarily urban based. Members also include a few dozen people from neighboring West African countries and about 20 from China. This diverse association thus represents a fundamental shift in the ways that knowledge of traditional medicine is exchanged in Niamey and in Niger in general, as it contrasts with

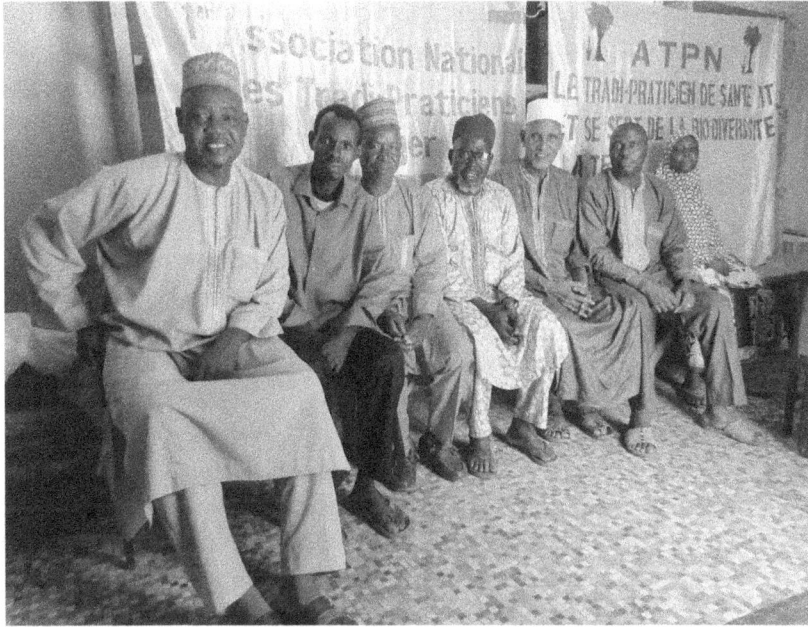

Figure 5.3. ATPN's Board of Directors. Photo by author.

the passing of knowledge through narrow family lines that has long been the tradition in Niger. ATPN provides members with opportunities to exchange medical knowledge and marketing strategies with fellow healers other than their parents, who represent all the ethnic groups and regions of Niger. This usually transpires at small, informal meetings at regional offices or in members' compounds, though ATPN did hold one national-level meeting in 2010 and is planning another. Indeed, ATPN is contributing to an emerging and evolving transethnic traditional medicine. There are no formal ethnic-based traditional healers' associations in Niger.

The directors regard building the reputation of traditional medicine and healers as a core part of ATPN's mission. This is partly to counteract exponentially rising popularity of informal-sector street sales of pharmaceutical drugs. They proudly emphasized that they are a state-registered NGO, and that the government and its Ministry of Public Health support them. Members are issued laminated ATPN picture identification or membership cards. According to the directors, police do not disturb healers who present ATPN membership cards that help to confirm their legitimacy. In contrast, police sometimes harass healers without cards by accusing them of selling illicit drugs. Furthermore, traditional healers show their membership cards to clients to enhance their credibility. Members of ATPN who use packaging put ATPN on their labels, though I as learned from long study of other products sold on street in Niamey, anyone can put any label on anything.

The Nigérien traditional healers' organization's decision to affiliate itself with the state, even loosely as an NGO, was a risky one. After all, Nigériens are deeply mistrustful of their government and its support of biomedicine. The reality is that ATPN receives minimal support and recognition from the Nigérien government, and no funding. One important exception to this is the annual African Traditional Medicine Day that was initiated by the WHO in 2003 to valorize traditional medicine and is cosponsored by Niger's Ministry of Public Health. The event is a multiday affair. For example, in 2019 it began with an opening ceremony in the primary conference room of Stade Général Seyni Kountché (Niger's national football stadium) featuring speeches by WHO representatives, the Minister of Public Health, ATPN board members, and others, before continuing with a 10-day exposition of traditional medicine on the grounds of the Grande Mosquée Kadhafi de Niamey—the city's most important mosque. The placement of the exposition at Niamey's Friday Mosque signaled that Nigérien traditional plant medicines are compatible with Islam. This was critical to building trust in traditional medicine in a predominantly Muslim country.

Beyond affiliating with ATPN, Nigérien traditional healers manipulate material culture, including the ways that they transport and display medicines as well as the medicines themselves, in ways creatively calculated to overcome patients' mistrust. However, it is not always clear what will earn the trust of clients, and traditional healers perceive that clients' perspectives are changing, particularly with the rapid rise of itinerant pharmaceutical healers. Hence traditional healers are adapting the material culture of their trade. The material culture of most traditional healers is rustic. Most healers carry their plant medicines in burlap bags or repurposed plastic rice sacks, or display them in bundles on standard pushcarts, or spread them out on thatched mats on the ground. Some traditional healers simply cannot afford more expensive tools of the trade or to rent a market stall, but others choose simple accoutrements to project down-to-earth personas. For example, a plastic sack-carrying 60-year-old Hausa healer explained to me, "I can afford a pushcart and the megaphone that other healers use, and I have nice clothes at home not like these old, dusty ones that you see me wearing. But I want clients to know that I am a man of the earth and not think that I am only in it for the money." In contrast, other traditional healers work from fixed locations and can offer patients shade and chairs to sit down. A few use automobiles and tables to set up extensive daily displays. These higher-end, temporary traditional medicine pharmacies typically use loudspeakers and large (5- by 10- meter) professionally painted cloth banners that list the ailments that they treat.

Traditional healers are also adapting the packaging of their medicines to build consumer confidence and increase their profits. The longstanding and still most common method of dispensing plant medicine is to simply wrap the leaves, twigs, or bark in a piece of scrap paper and hand it to the customer with oral instructions about dosages and applications such as mixing it with tea, rubbing the mixture on the body, or burning the plants and inhaling the smoke. In recent years, some traditional healers have begun adopting biomedical marketing strategies—namely, they are now packaging traditional medicine. Typically, this packaging is very crude, consisting of a sealed, clear plastic bag with a typed or handwritten note describing uses and sometimes

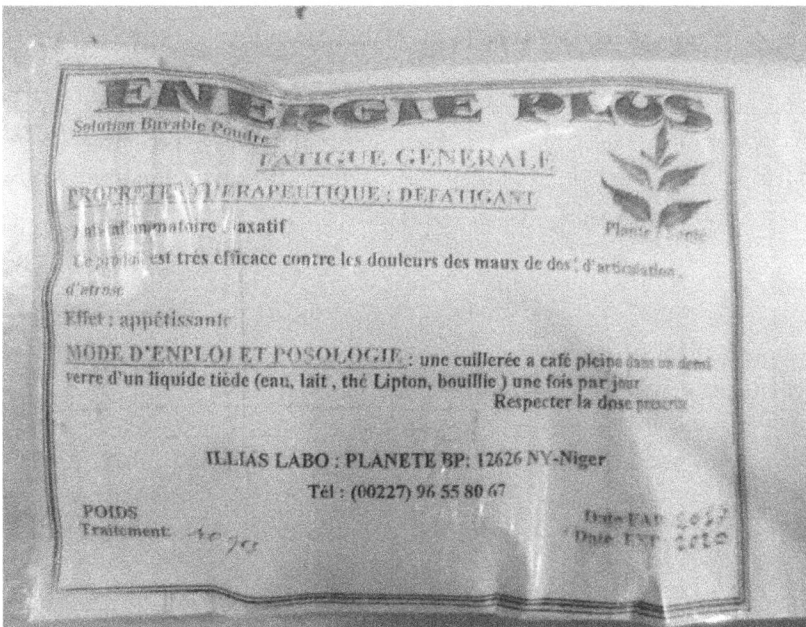

Figure 5.4. Packaged traditional medicine. Photo by author.

the ingredients. In a small but steadily rising number of cases, industrial packaging is used, made in Niger and in neighboring countries. For the same quantity of plant medicine, vendors can raise the price by 50 times or more in some cases, if it is industrially packaged versus sold off a mat and passed to a client in a piece of paper. In another example, many traditional healers are now advertising their medicines through social media, particularly Facebook and WhatsApp.

Traditional healers continue to thrive in Niamey by regularly adapting to local needs to overcome multiple sources of mistrust. They offer convenient, affordable access to health care while appealing to pride in local heritage. Traditional healers of Niamey enjoy an advantage over their counterparts in rural Niger where 75 percent of Nigériens live in that most people in Niamey have very limited access to the bush—the source of plant medicines.[6] Traditional healers and Islamic healers—the subject of the following discussion— both rely on tradition while adapting adeptly to contemporary times.

### Islamic Healers of Niamey Overcoming Mistrust

Islamic healers in Niamey seek to appeal to the Muslim piety of their patients to earn their trust. Several of Islamic healers I interviewed quoted the Prophet Muhammad, "Allah did not send down to earth a disease without having at the same time sending down its remedy," or more simply, "For every illness, Allah created a remedy," and some have written the phrase on their shops. They argue that Islamic medicine is appropriate for Muslims because it has been made by Muslims according to Islamic tradition and laws. One of Kelley Sams's (2017, 1112) participants described in detail the attraction of Islamic medicine, "These are made for Muslims. By Muslims for Muslims, and they are stronger than anything that you can buy made by Atheists. Maybe for Christians you have your own medicine, but for Muslims, this is what we have that is ours. It comes from the same place that our religion comes from . . . It comes from the direction we face when we pray." Islamic healers highlight the sacred qualities of their medicine, often referring to them as *coranisé* (Qur'anized or holy)—for example, *miel coranisé* (holy honey). They, like traditional healers, regularly assert that their medicines are natural and plant-based, though they do not use the term *bio* (organic) nearly as often as traditional healers do. I overhead Elhadji Mamansani, a 50-year-old Hausa man who opened an Islamic medicine shop in 2018, summarize the

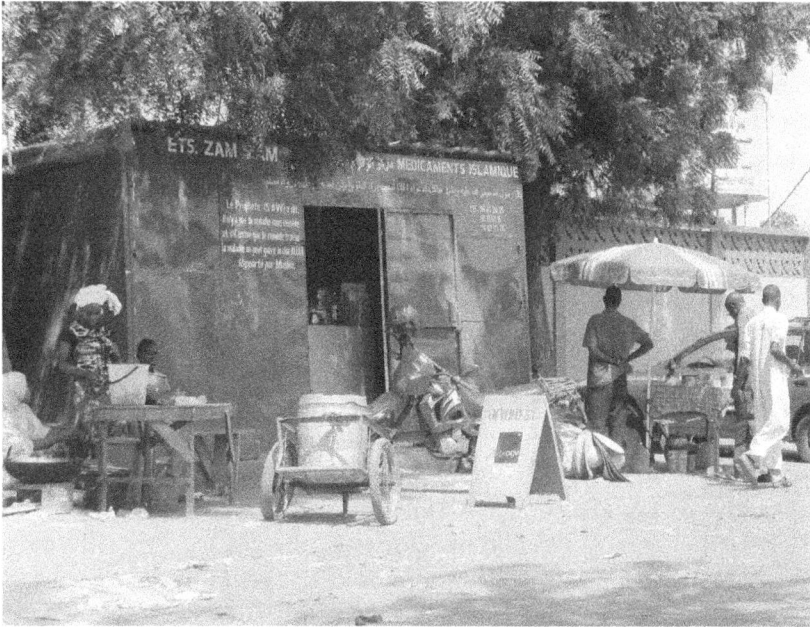

Figure 5.5. Islamic medicine shop. Photo by author.

advantages of his medicines to a patient: "My products are plant-based, they are not toxic, they are less expensive and efficacious. They are referenced in the Holy Qur'an."

Therapies for a full range of illnesses of naturalistic origins as well as illnesses of supernatural origins, including Islamic methods for preventing jinn, witchcraft, and sorcery attacks and exorcising jinn are offered by Islamic healers (see Table I.1). They emphasize that their exorcism methods are morally superior to those of Nigérien traditional religions that involve cajoling and flattering named local spirits. Furthermore, Islamic healers in Niger offer several medicines that are quasi-panaceas, many of which are "food-medicines"; that is, foods that have both nutritional and medicinal value. They are taken prophylactically to maintain health and retroactively to treat many conditions. The five most important "food-medicines," all of which are mentioned in the Qur'an, are honey, ajwa dates, olive oil, ginger, and black cumin seeds.[7] In addition, most Islamic healers in Niamey sell Zam Zam water. This holy water from a well in Mecca just 20 meters east of the Kaaba is considered a virtual panacea.

Islamic healers use symbols of Islamic piety as part of their social and personal identities and to project authority. They wear Muslim attire; namely, male healers wear flowing gowns and skullcaps, and female healers don their own type of loose-fitting gowns and layers of headscarves and veils that cover most of their skin.[8] When the men are not interacting with patients or arranging and rearranging their medicine displays in their boutiques or on their pushcarts, they typically sit on benches whispering prayers while fingering prayer beads or reading the Qur'an and other Islamic books. While these acts serve to bring them closer to God, they also make their piety visible to others, which helps to reinforce their seriousness and legitimacy. Islamic healers in Niamey are committed to community engagement and pray together with neighbors.

A wide range of other strategies are used by Islamic healers to earn the trust of patients. They offer relative *convenience* as their shops are usually open eight hours a day, seven days a week, except at Muslim prayer times. Islamic healers exude *seriousness* while also being *friendly* with patients and attentive to norms of greeting and everyday conversation. This helps them forge connections while projecting knowledge and focus. They patiently show *respect* and *empathy* for their clients and listen carefully to them. Some of these consultations last 30 minutes or more, but most interactions are perfunctory because clients have already decided what medication they want before they arrive. Islamic healers seek a balance between sharing medical knowledge with their patients and offering explanations of their diagnoses and therapies on the one hand and keeping some of their knowledge hidden on the other. Because most Islamic healers work in roadside boutiques, they can offer more confidentiality and privacy to patients than traditional healers and itinerant pharmaceutical healers who primarily work on the street. The very fact that they have shops differentiates them most other informal-sector healers and communicates a serious level of commitment.

Islamic healers of Niamey change and adapt in response to the strong influence of Northern Nigeria. Muslim practice and teaching in Northern Nigeria—especially in Kano, the cultural and Islamic capital of the region— have an enormous impact on Muslim religiosity in Niger. Trends in Northern Nigerian Islam tend to become trends in Nigérien Islam with a lag time of a few years. For example, the Salafist-inspired Izala reform movement was established in Jos, Nigeria, in 1978 and rapidly took hold across Northern Nigeria before arriving in Niger, where it took much longer to gain popularity, in late 1980s.[9] This includes trends in Islamic medicine. In the case of Islamic medicine, the lag time lasted decades, but an important transformation that

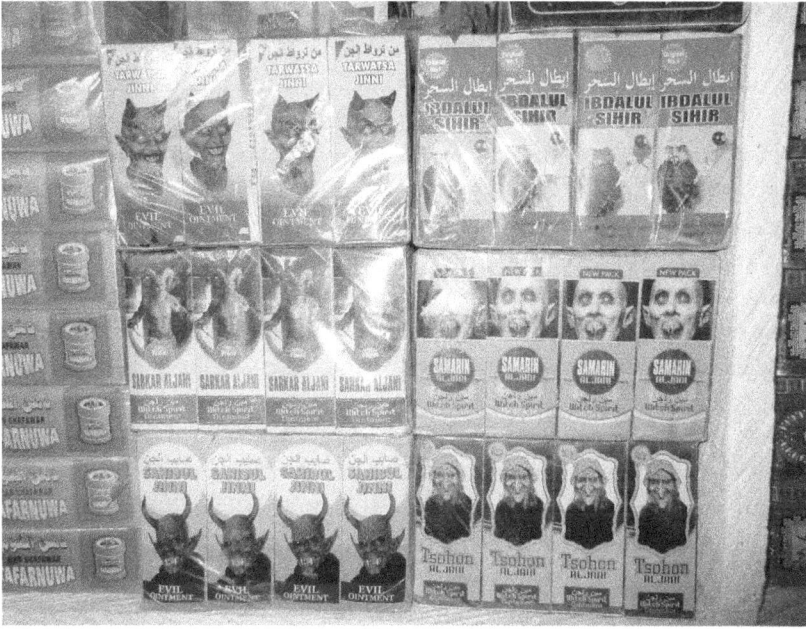

Figure 5.6. Interior of Islamic medicine shop. Photo by author.

is currently transpiring warrants some discussion because it suggests where
Niamey may be headed.

Until recently in Niger and Northern Nigeria, almost all Islamic healers were Islamic leaders and scholars who also practiced medicine. They are
referred to with the generic Arabic term as marabout as well as many other
honorifics in local languages, such as *malam* (sing.) and *malamai* (pl.) in
Hausa. Beginning in the late 1980s in Kano, Nigeria, some people began referring to themselves as "Islamic pharmacists" or "Islamic chemists." Initially,
these Islamic pharmacists were well-known scholars and authors of medical
books with advanced degrees in Islamic studies and Arabic. However, as their
popularity grew it became a lucrative business, leading to the "proliferation
of sub-standard Islamic medicines and incompetent practitioners . . . [and
casting] doubt on the credibility of genuine" pharmacists (Yahaya 2023, 202,
205). According to Alhassan (2022, 11), one of the first "modern Islamic
Health Centers" to open in Nigeria was the Sangarib Trado-Medical Center
in Kano in 1988. By "modern Islamic Health Center," Alhassan meant that
they offered packaged Islamic medicine, in contrast with the longstanding

methods used by marabouts of dispensing medicine in scrap paper or repurposed cans and jars. The proprietor of Sangarib Trado-Medical Center was a well-known Islamic scholar who also studied medicine in Mecca while on the hajj, but he thought it presumptuous to put "Islamic" in the name of his medical center. By 1992, medical centers and pharmacies of Kano began using the term "Islamic" in their names and have ever since. Some of Kano's Islamic medical centers (and some of the pharmacies too), are multiroom complexes with waiting rooms; consultation rooms; rooms where plant medicines are dried, compounded, and packaged; rooms with Islamic medical books; and guest rooms to accommodate in-patient services. The in-patient service most in demand was *ruk'ya*, or the exorcism of jinn (Alhassan 2022, 14).[10]

Islamic medical centers, pharmacies, and chemists (at some point, the latter became the most commonly used term) have proliferated in Kano and in all of the cities of Northern Nigeria. A simple Google Maps search of "Kano Islamic pharmacies" yielded more than 200 results. (Kano has a population of about 5 million people.) The most significant change in Islamic medicine in Kano, Alhassan (2022, 15) argued, was that "The emergence of modern Islamic health centers led to a shift where[by] these health centers overtook the *Mallam* [sic.] practitioners" by 2012. Today's Islamic chemists of Kano creatively use social media—especially Facebook, TikTok, WhatsApp, and YouTube—and "influencer marketing" such as hiring Islamic scholars, celebrities, Kannywood film stars, and musicians to create a sense of community, build their reputations, and advertise their services and products (Yahaya 2023, 211).

In Niamey, where healers did not begin calling themselves "Islamic pharmacists" and opening "Islamic pharmacies" until about 2015, Islamic pharmacists are a long way from "overtaking" marabout or *malamai* healers. The "traditional" Islamic healers of Niamey and their locally sourced Islamic medicines are generally trusted. The new "modern" Islamic pharmacists and their imported, packaged medicines are viewed with considerable skepticism by people in Niamey. Some Islamic pharmacists are lifelong Islamic scholars, but others are essentially entrepreneurs who are learning Islamic medicine on the fly. Many of the Islamic pharmacies of Niamey are stocked primarily with boxed medicines made in Kano that are designed either to repel djinn, witchcraft, or sorcery attacks or to exorcise djinn that have possessed victims. (The most common other products are very similar to those found in the pharmacies of Kano and elsewhere in Northern Nigeria such as honey, ginger, dates, olive oil, black cumin seeds, and Zam Zam water.) Parallel to

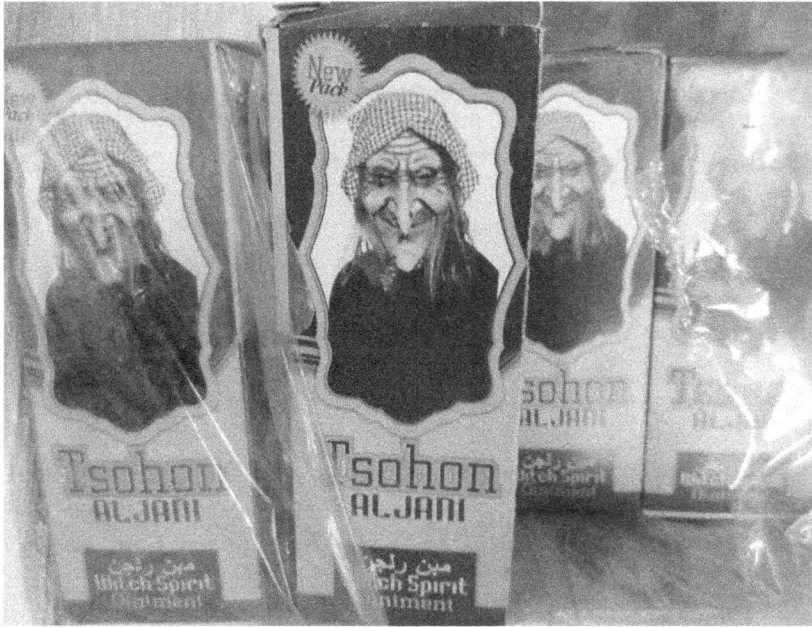

Figure 5.7. Islamic anti-witch medicine. Photo by author.

15 years ago in Kano where "some people in the public consider[ed] *ruk'ya* healing of modern Islamic health centers similar to *bori* [and] consider[ed] it as a new way of having intercession with the spirits" (Alhassan 2022, 16), many people in Niamey today are puzzled by this emphasis on jinn. They are also not sure whether these medicines work with spirits of local traditional religions. Islamic healers of Niamey explain to clients that Islam recognizes the existence of jinn, sorcery, and witchcraft, and they emphatically tell them that their *Islamic* medicines are designed to deter and expel them.

There are now about 100 Islamic pharmacists operating in Niamey, according to my interviews. A 40-year-old Zarma man who opened an Islamic pharmacy in the Yantala neighborhood of Niamey explained, "We are a Muslim country, so we do not need to ask for authorization to open an Islamic pharmacy." Only about 20 of them have signage that includes the word "Islamic"; the remainder have no signage. Malam Hassane, an Islamic healer, explained why he has not bothered to erect a sign in a way that I found representative: "I have operated my little shop in this neighborhood for 25 years. Everyone in the neighborhood knows where I am, so I do not need a sign." A simple Google

Maps search of "Niamey Islamic pharmacies" yielded only four results, one of which was a bookstore, Librarie Islamique Al-Kahf. As far as I know, there are no Islamic medical centers in Niamey that offer in-patient therapy, such as jinn exorcisms, only one-room pharmacies. However, Islamic pharmacists and pharmacies of Niamey offer products that resonate with the Nigérien ethos of self-care. Namely, they offer products—boxed and shrink-wrapped plant medicines—for do-it-yourself djinn exorcisms at home, in contrast with the multiday *ruk'ya* of the Islamic medical centers of Northern Nigeria. This illustrates one way that these healers work to gain patients' trust by ensuring that their products meet local needs. While predicting the future is risky—especially for a place with intense uncertainty like Niger—I suggest that Islamic medicine and pharmacists will continue to expand rapidly in Niamey.

Islamic healers of Niamey also change and adapt in response to competition from rivals in other medical sectors. They position themselves vis-à-vis traditional and biomedical healers but largely ignore them. Instead, they mostly rest on the belief they view as self-evident, that Islamic medicine is most appropriate and suitable for Muslims. However, Islamic healers, especially the emerging "modern" Islamic pharmacists, of Niamey are using packaged medicines, which in some ways is a response to pharmaceutical packaging, and some are using social media—Facebook, TikTok, WhatsApp, and YouTube—to advertise their medicines in part because they know traditional healers are too.

Islamic healers creatively manipulate various dimensions of the material culture of their medical practice to overcome the mistrust of their patients. Most Islamic healers of Niamey work in small shops. Their boutiques are typically attached to mosques where they sell Islamic prayer rugs, prayer beads, skullcaps, the Qur'an, and other Islamic books alongside Islamic medicine. This communicates to customers that all these items are important to being Muslim. Others operate stand-alone shops. A few of the Islamic medicine shops of Niamey feature signage, usually including both Arabic and French. The use of Arabic confers Islamic legitimacy, while the use of French is practical as it is the written language that Nigériens are most likely to understand. A minority of Islamic healers in Niamey work on foot and use pushcarts that are like those used by traditional healers and biomedical healers. However, many shop owners are mobile on Thursday evenings, the regular time of *wa'izi* (Islamic preaching) in Niger. They converge at *wa'izi* venues—typically at mosques that have space in front of them—and set up mats and small tables on the periphery to sell their Islamic medicines and other Muslim goods. Dogo, a 60-year-old Hausa man, earns a living largely by selling milk and honey once a week at *wa'izi*.

Islamic healers of Niamey increasingly use packaged medicines to overcome patients' mistrust, with mixed results. Like traditional healers, many Islamic healers, especially the older *malamai*, also dispense medicine in simple ways, such as in scrap paper and repurposed cans, jars, and bottles to promote local authenticity. Today, many, especially the generally younger Islamic pharmacists, are using primarily packaged medicines. Several Islamic healers explained that patients have confidence that packaged medicines with listed expiration dates are sanitary and protected and not exposed to dust and the sun like those of many Islamic healers in Niger. The provenance of Islamic medicines in Niamey—especially of the packaged varieties—is primarily foreign. Cheiffou, a middle-aged Zarma healer, explained the appeal of imported Islamic medicines, in ways that were representative of other Islamic healers I interviewed: "Increasing numbers of my patients think that Islamic medicines of foreign Islamic countries—especially Saudi Arabia—are more powerful than our own. This is why I display them prominently, though I have plenty of Islamic medicines made in Niger too. When they see Arabic on the labels, they are convinced that it is authentic Islamic medicine." Arabic script carries weight in Niger, even though very few Nigériens—less than 5 percent, including Islamic healers—can read the various forms of modern Arabic used on medical packaging.

The boxed and shrink-wrapped medicines made in Kano are a particularly interesting subset of imported Islamic medicines in Niamey. As highlighted earlier, these products, which are designed either to repel jinn, witchcraft, or sorcery attacks or to exorcise jinn that have possessed victims, dominate the inventory of several Islamic medicine shops in Niamey. Clearly some Islamic healers of Niamey have clients who are interested in these new medicines, though I have also highlighted that there is considerable mistrust of them among Nigériens. The writing on the labels always includes some Arabic but is mostly in Hausa and English. The labels specify what the contents treat, directions for use, and expiration dates. They often indicate that the contents are "100% Natural" but do not indicate the specific plant medicines included. The contents of these boxes are sealed plastic bags of powdered plant medicines. For example, Sayful Jinni's box claims verbatim that "It cures jinn and spirit attack, fear, charm, doubting or jinn that do marry human (both men and women). It also cures women menstrual problems, miscarriages, bad

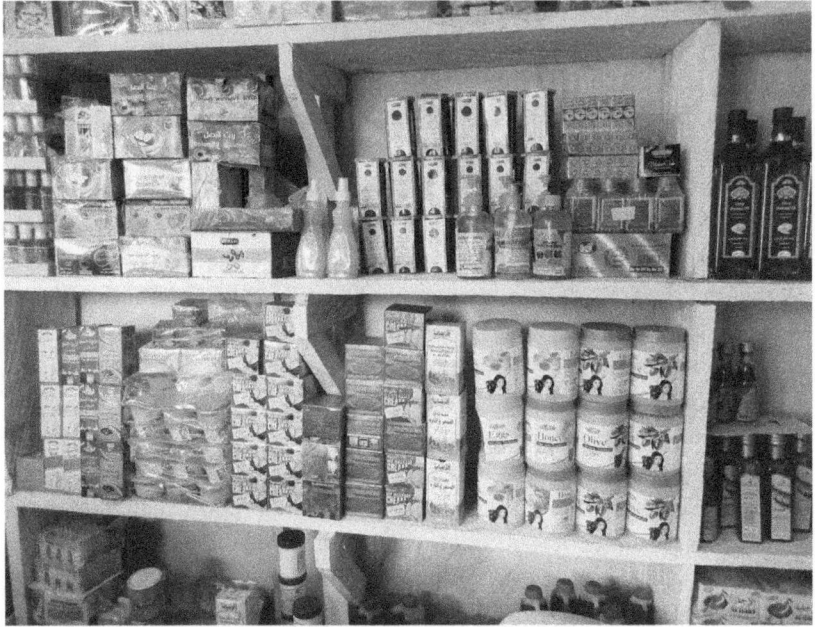

Figure 5.8. Interior of Islamic medicine shop. Photo by author.

dreams and other evil related illnesses both hidden & exposed" and directs patients to "Rub the medicine two times daily morning and evening." Islamic healers typically carry medicines that are purported to treat a very broad range of illnesses, as I pointed out in my discussion of "food-medicines."

I argue that the most striking element of the labels is the imagery of "evil spirits," in part because very few Nigériens can read English or Hausa.[11] Islamic chemists of Kano have creatively adapted—or perhaps just lifted— images of spirits, demons, zombies, and witches from the global popular culture of horror films for their labels. They depict jinn and devils as White.[12] I witnessed the aftermath of the opening of new Islamic medicine shop of Niamey in 2018. Though anecdotal, the events I observed and the discussion that ensued with nearby witnesses illustrate the typical reactions of initial mistrust of these packaged, anti-evil spirit medicines that healers must overcome. A couple of weeks after the shop opened a group of children picked through a pile of trash near the shop. They shrieked in terror when they saw the images of demons on discarded medicine boxes and ran away. One boy, however, was bold enough to pick up one of the boxes, and he was summoned by a small group of middle-aged men whom I know gathered nearby for conversation who had heard the commotion. The men were dismayed by the image of a menacing, muscle-bound humanoid with horns on his head. One man said, "Spirits should not be depicted, this will only attract them and anger them." His friend agreed, and added, "What is this stuff, is it even Islamic medicine?" Yet by one year later, a couple of men in this group had tried the anti-evil spirit medicine, but only after friends had shared it with them. When I asked the shop's proprietor about this, he explained, "These are powerful Islamic medicines from Kano. Yes, the pictures are scary because jinn are frightening."

Like traditional healers, Islamic healers of Niamey provide convenient, relatively affordable treatments for the full range of illnesses recognized by Nigériens. They can offer more privacy than traditional healers and pharmaceutical healers. Given the "re-Islamization" of Niger in recent years, "traditional" Islamic healers who sell mostly local, unpackaged Islamic medicines are generally trusted. In contrast, Nigériens have reacted with skepticism but also curiosity to the emergence of Islamic pharmacists and packaged Islamic medicines. These newer practitioners must work hard to overcome Nigériens' mistrust. Not only have traditional healers and Islamic healers competed for patients for more than a century in Niamey, but both have also had to contend with the rise of itinerant pharmaceutical vending over the past 25 years.

## Itinerant Biomedical Healers of
## Niamey Overcoming Mistrust

Itinerant pharmaceutical healers of Niamey draw on the promise of modernity and science to overcome patients' mistrust. They are most commonly called *akwaku*, a Hausa term.[13] Since *akwaku* began operating 25 years ago and especially in the last decade, their subaltern health innovations that draw from global markets and are adapted to local cultural and economic conditions have enabled them to become the perhaps the most popular source of medicines in Niamey. The rise of the *akwaku* is not a simple matter, given that Nigériens have deeply mistrusted biomedicine for decades. *Akwaku* offer biomedical drugs for a full range of illnesses of naturalistic origin. (See Table I.1.) They do not claim that they can cure illnesses of supernatural origin, although they assert that they can alleviate some of the symptoms of supernatural attacks. As such, they present themselves and their medicines primarily as a convenient, affordable, and pragmatic alternative to formal-sector biomedicine. *Akwaku* also know that they compete for patients in the informal sector because traditional and Islamic healers also treat illnesses of naturalistic origin.

*Akwaku* are simultaneously healers and entrepreneurs, though they identify primarily as the latter. As healers they voluntarily or upon request offer diagnoses and suggest specific pharmaceuticals to treat illnesses. In most cases, they simply sell whatever clients request. A recent journalistic account concludes that, "In Niger, unregulated medicine is 'sold like sweets'" (Observer 2018). At times they genuinely care about the health of their clients, whereas at other times they care primarily about their own incomes. Clearly, they aim to please. As one consumer explained, "If you ask *akwaku* if they have medicine for a particular illness, they will always say 'yes,' no matter what." They want repeat customers. They care about their reputations and do not want clients spreading rumors that they are charlatans. However, they are also aware that they must take risks to maximize sales even when they are not confident that their recommendations will help clients. In familiar-sounding words, one young Fulani man offered his appraisal: "*Akwaku* neither want their clients to die nor do they want to completely heal them because either way they will lose clients."

*Akwaku* narratives reveal that they consider themselves first and foremost as successful entrepreneurs. *Akwaku* means "clerk" in Hausa, though I have only occasionally heard it used to refer clerks who sell products other than medicines. Two-thirds explained that they chose this profession for economic reasons; that is, to make a lot of money relatively easily due to the high markups on the drugs they buy cheaply from wholesalers and the presence of many clients in most neighborhoods of the city.[14] The profession is relatively lucrative. The 60 *akwaku* in the sample reported earning an average of nearly 4,000 CFA daily (8 USD)—a handsome sum relative to the 1.5 USD average daily per capita income in Niger. Some of the *akwakus'* choices indicate that their main focus is on earning money. For example, before creating my interview questions, I noticed that *akwaku* commonly sell cigarettes, so I decided to ask them about it. Fifty-five of the 60 *akwaku* interviewed sell cigarettes. Most explained that this was simply a way to earn more money or that their clients request them. One *akwaku* explained, "I use cigarettes as a lure. I initially attract customers with cigarettes, then they see my medicines and sometimes buy some." Many other *akwaku* offered similar explanations. Those who do not sell cigarettes said that they made this choice because cigarettes are dangerous for health. Like the *akwaku*, many U.S. pharmacies also continue to sell cigarettes (Lowes 2018).

*Akwaku* project authority even though many have a narrow base of knowledge about health, illnesses, and healing. In contrast with the long apprenticeships of traditional healers and most Islamic healers, and the standardized education and certification of formal-sector biomedical professionals, *akwaku* build their expertise through daily informal discussions with a wide range of people and through the diffuse general knowledge of pharmaceuticals in Niamey, where almost everyone thinks they know something about pharmaceuticals. One needs only the capital to buy some medicines and a sack to carry them to get started. An *akwaku*, expressing a majority opinion among the group, explained that "When in doubt I most often ask questions of wholesalers, they are the most knowledgeable experts on the drugs." Many *akwaku* explained that they trust the wholesalers because they see all the new drugs coming into Niamey and have made substantial investments in their trade. The next most common way of building knowledge is through discussions with fellow *akwaku* and others that have experience including, in some cases, professional formal-sector pharmacists. *Akwaku* also decipher the uses of drugs by viewing the photographic images on many package labels. These images often highlight parts of the body that the drugs are purported to target and heal and are designed to appeal to nonliterate audiences. Only a minority indicated that they learn about the content, usages, and dosages of their products by reading packaging labels because three-quarters of *akwaku* are nonliterate. A few state that the uses of many of their drugs are simply "common knowledge" in Niamey, or that they already knew about them from prior experience as consumers. Fifty of the sixty *akwaku* in my sample learned their craft in Niamey, typically in their own neighborhoods.

Itinerant pharmaceutical healers of Niamey face many physical, intellectual, and social challenges in their work. Most walk the hot, dusty, uneven streets of Niamey eight hours daily carrying their medicine towers. Those with pushcarts have an only slightly easier job. Their energy and initiative signify that they are regular Nigériens of the same socioeconomic milieu as most of their customers. They typically wear Western attire such as jeans and polo shirts, though some wear simple Muslim clothing, which becomes dusty and sweat-stained by midday. This clothing choice signals their modernity, which they try to project onto their medicines. Furthermore, *akwaku* must convince patients that they have knowledge of ailments, diseases, and medicines. They also need to memorize the prices of dozens of products.

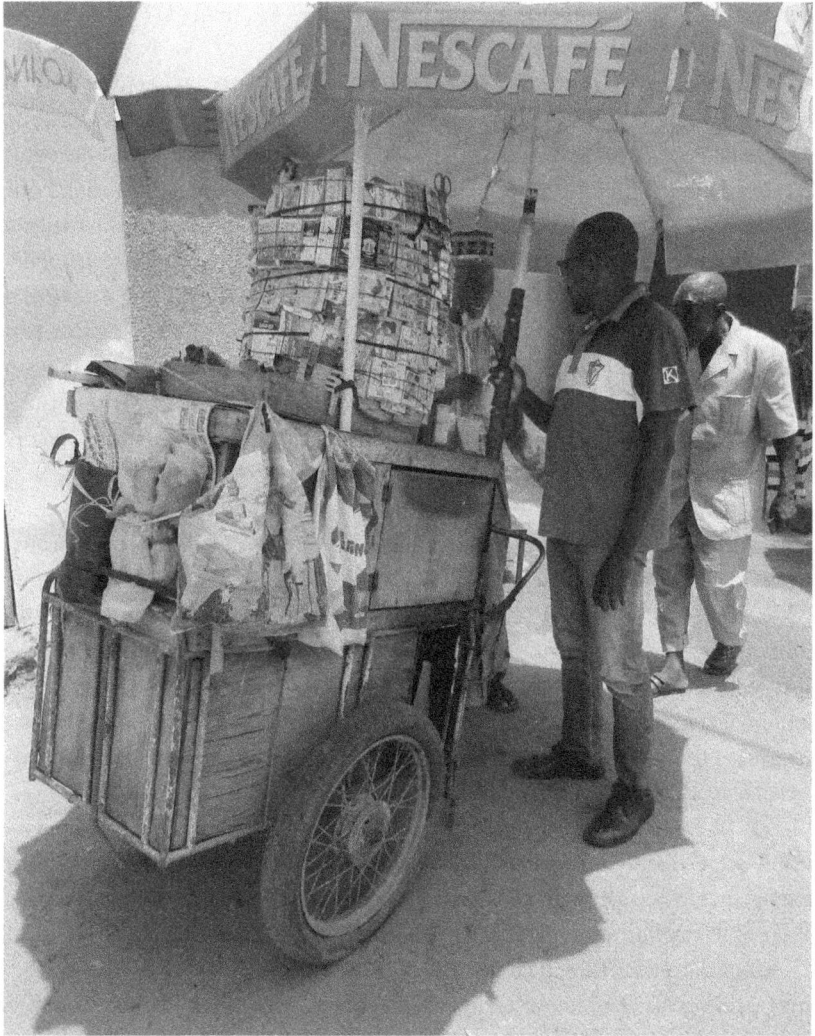

Figure 5.9. Itinerant pharmaceutical vendor with medical tower on pushcart. Photo by author.

*Akwaku* generate trust in their version of biomedical practice through the ways that they present themselves and their products and interact with clients to produce new meanings for pharmaceuticals. The success of the *akwaku* depends, in large part, on their social skills. The social and power distances between *akwaku* and their clients are far narrower than the distance between formal-sector health professional and their patients, and *akwaku* seek to capitalize on this to earn trust in their products and knowledge. They typically walk standardized routes through their own neighborhoods and develop some loyal customers. Some make house calls for regular clients. *Akwaku* exchange greetings with and treat patients respectfully and speak with them in common local languages such as Zarma, Hausa, Fulfulde, and Tamashek— contributing to patients' trust in them. These behaviors are what is expected of trusted friends and neighbors and they contribute to feelings of trust. They are friendly and eager to answer questions about medicines and diseases. They do not question or criticize their clients' health concepts or decisions. Despite the risk, some extend credit to long-time customers.

The *akwaku* offer Nigériens *affordable, convenient, liberating* access to pharmaceuticals on familiar local terms. Because they typically sell generic pharmaceuticals made in the Global South and offer dosing flexibility—they regularly sell one pill at a time—*akwaku* vend their drugs for a small fraction of the prices demanded by formal-sector pharmacies that primarily sell name-brand pharmaceuticals manufactured in France and only full bottles of medicines or full courses of treatment. The prices charged by *awkaku* for their medicines are comparable to those asked by traditional healers and generally slightly lower than the prices of Islamic medicines for treating similar problems. *Akwaku* make themselves available throughout daylight hours and into the evening. Nigériens in Niamey can find them within minutes and usually do not have to wait to speak with them for more than a few minutes if at all.

Furthermore, the pharmaceutical drugs dispensed by the *akwaku* carry the *hope of quick healing*. Almost all of the medicines sold by the *akwaku* can be ingested immediately. This contrasts with often hours-long waiting lines at formal-sector health facilities, and after visiting hospitals and clinics Nigériens must travel to pharmacies and wait some more for service. The *akwaku*'s pills that can be swallowed on the spot offer a practical, time-saving alternative to many of the plant medicines sold by traditional and Islamic healers that often require time-consuming preparation and administration, such as inhaling incense or taking long herbal baths over the course of several days. The drugs provided by *akwaku* "break the hegemony of professionals and enable people to help themselves" (van der Geest and Whyte 1989, 348). This is appreciated by Nigériens, many of whom prefer self-care with the guidance of therapy management groups. *Akwaku* also provide the privacy and anonymity that Nigérien patients value but is not offered in most formal-sector hospitals and clinics. For example, I observed several *akwaku* selling abortifacient pharmaceuticals even though abortions are culturally taboo as well as illegal in Niger unless a licensed physician determines that the mother's life is at risk (Cooper 2019, 286).

Abdoulrazack, a young Zarma *akwaku*, shared an astute conclusion that was representative of comments made by other *akwaku* with whom I spoke: "Even if patients do not trust me, they trust the medicines that I sell." Abdoulrazack's comment illustrates the key argument made by Whyte, van der Geest, and Hardon (2002, 1, original emphasis) argue that medicines are "the material *things* of therapy." The key to "the charm of medicines" is their "concreteness," they "are the hard core of therapy and what it is that sets them apart from other forms of healing" (van der Geest and Whyte 1989, 345). One of the reasons that pharmaceuticals are so desirable is that many believe that they have the power of healing in themselves and "even removed from their medical context they retain a potential connection to it . . . with medical doctors who prescribe them, with laboratories that produce them, with medical science that forms their ultimate ground" (ibid., 359). The *akwaku* enable Nigériens to "enjoy the fruits of medical expertise without the inconvenience of actually having to go to the doctor" (ibid., 359). Pharmaceuticals meet an urgent need for which theoretically there is unlimited demand so long as people trust them and the people who sell them.

*Akwaku* of Niamey use a relatively uniform material culture to display their pharmaceuticals. Most—34 of 60 in the sample—sell their products from cylindrical wooden towers that are about one meter in height. These are carried atop their heads or shoulders. They strap drug packages around their cylinders with thick rubber bands that typically completely cover the wood, to create visually striking mobile pharmacies. Most also hand carry waist-high wooden stools on which they put their towers so that their customers can look at their goods at eye level. Others—12 of 60—put their cylinders on wooden and metal pushcarts with two bicycle tires that typically include umbrellas. Ten others set up their carts or tables at fixed roadside spots, while four vend from small boutiques.

Despite the general similarity of their medicine towers, *akwaku* take great care to personalize their displays. Each *akwaku* creates unique color combinations through arrangements of drug packaging and particular patterns for using rubber bands to keep them in place. They use empty packages if necessary to ensure that all parts of their towers are covered, presumably to

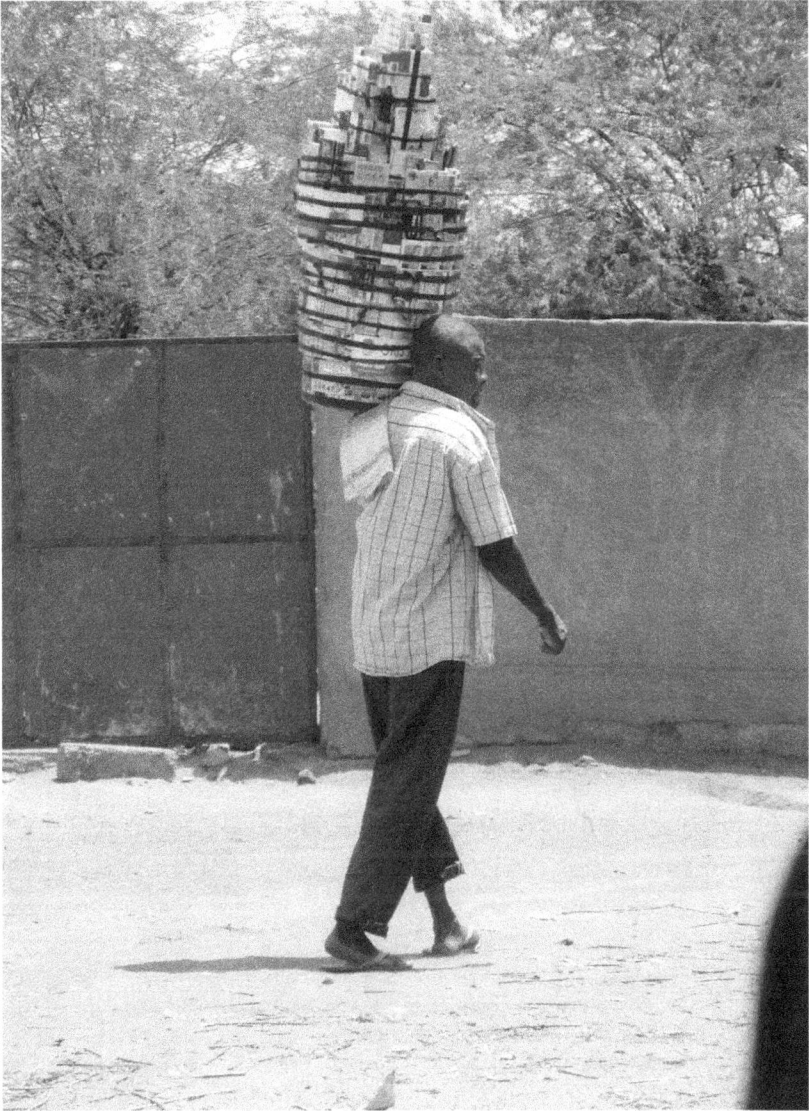

Figure 5.10. Itinerant pharmaceutical vendor with medical tower on shoulder. Photo by author.

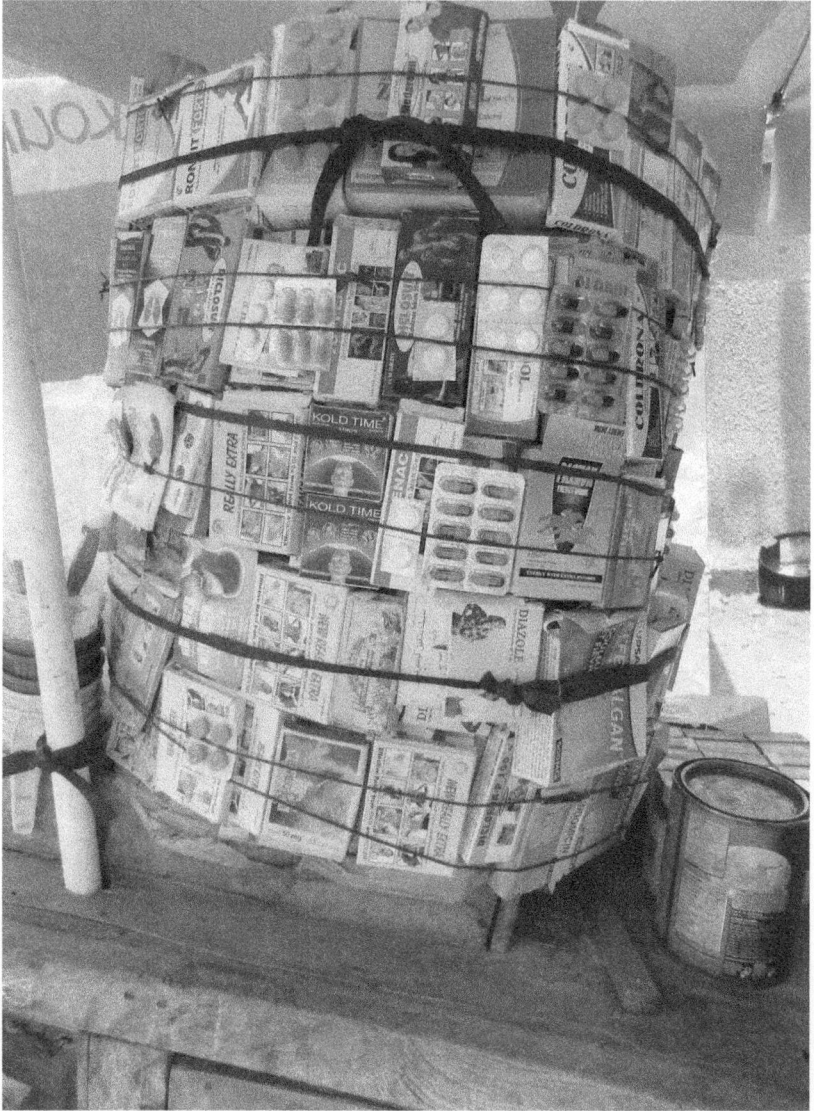

Figure 5.11. Pharmaceutical drugs on medicine tower. Photo by author.

impress on potential clients that they are well stocked. *Akwaku* with pushcarts have more space to work with to accentuate their businesses with umbrellas, decals, and additional products such as kola nuts and dates—items traditionally exchanged by friends and distributed at Muslim baby-naming ceremonies and weddings in Niger. The inclusion of kola nuts and dates further integrates them in valued community practices and thus helps build trust.

*Akwaku* prefer marketing pharmaceuticals in blister packs over bottles because blister packs can more easily be strapped to wooden cylinders. Furthermore, *akwaku* can display more blister packs than bottles, and the blister packs usually have more colorful images than bottles do. A young *akwaku* explained another key benefit of blister packs: "They are ideal for selling medicine. Nigériens like to see the colors and shapes of my medicines just like they do with traditional medicine. My patients can see the drugs, but they are protected and sanitary in the blister packs." This is another example of healers adapting to local desires to help build patients' trust.

The local nomenclature for drugs and some of the ways that drugs are used further illustrate the indigenization of biomedicine through the *akwaku*. The most common drugs are referred to by *akwaku* and customers with abbreviated nicknames, such as para for paracetamol, ibu for ibuprophen, and amoxy for amoxycillin. The same is true of common diseases; for example, palu for *paludisme* (malaria). The people of Niamey have also created names for the popular drugs in local languages. For example, Really Extra is commonly known as *dori haku* (Zarma for "eight illnesses") in reference to the eight photographic images on its packaging of the pain in eight parts of the body it is purported to alleviate. Many of the pain-killing and anti-inflammatory medicines sold by *akwaku* contain caffeine are known as "anti-tiredness medicine" in Niamey—*maganin gajiya* and *hana kwana* in Hausa, *farga safari* in Zarma, and *missile* in French. The renaming of medicines frames them in local, familiar terms, contributing to patients' trust in them.

The flourishing *akwaku* sector in Niamey that originated 25 years ago involves creative adaptations to structural violence in a world in which health care is increasingly commoditized and privatized, where states and the "international community" have abdicated their responsibility to provide adequate health care to all people as a core human right. This was neither simple nor inevitable, as the *awkaku* have had to continuously confront Nigériens' long history of profound mistrust of biomedicine. The *awkaku* generate trust in their versions of biomedicine through the ways that they present themselves and their products on familiar local terms. Through diverting pharmaceuticals from the formal economy, the *akwaku* have significantly increased access to pharmaceuticals for millions of Nigériens and earn a good living in the process. *Akwaku* have made themselves trustworthy enough to emerge as key operators linking the globally dispersed production of pharmaceuticals with consumers on the streets of Niamey.

## Conclusion

The patient–healer relationship in Niamey is characterized by "mistrustful dependency" (Pasquini 2023). In Chapter 4, I emphasized this relationship from the perspective of patients, whereas in this chapter I have focused on this dyad from the perspective of healers who ultimately realize that Nigériens rely on them even when they mistrust them. They recognize the pervasive need for medicines in one of the world's poorest countries where people are constantly struggling with poor health and the state cannot provide health care for most of them due to structural adjustment and neoliberal reforms. Nevertheless, generalist traditional, Islamic, and biomedical healers who work on the streets of Niamey try hard to overcome their patients' mistrust. Healers of different medical sectors confront different sources of mistrust as well as some similar ones. Traditional healers confront more challenges than other healers, given that Muslim leaders and biomedical professionals have sought to undermine them for centuries and decades, respectively. I argue that this explains why, in the informal medical economies of Niamey, only traditional healers have established a formal association as a means of promoting their credibility.

Niamey's street healers attempt to draw patients in different ways, but also in overlapping ways and in response to one another and to formal-sector health care. They all seek to appeal to different Nigérien social identities and ideologies—cultural heritage, religion, and modernity—but share core strategies in their efforts to earn the trust of clients. Healers of all sectors adapt their work to the local context as an important way of overcoming mistrust. Street healers offer convenient and affordable access to health advice and medicines on cordial terms. Healers in Niamey's informal economy, especially traditional healers and *akwaku*, downplay social and power distances between themselves and their patients. Islamic healers prefer to project authority and knowledge but they, like traditional healers and *akwaku*, interact respectfully and patiently with clients. Street healers do not reprimand or speak down to patients. Healers in Niamey's informal economy choose to interact openly and kindly with patients in order to set themselves apart from formal-sector biomedical professionals. They are well aware of Nigériens' deep mistrust of hospitals, clinics, and pharmacies, and many have had negative experiences with them as well. In short, informal-sector healers of Niamey rely on "soft skills" to overcome patients' mistrust, including respect, empathy, listening, adaptability, and the use of persuasion rather than coercion. However, cultural competence among healers is differentiating. Some healers attract more patients than others because they are more socially skilled and charismatic than their rivals.

Street healers of Niamey stick with "tried and true" strategies while always looking for new ways to build trust and attract patients. Many traditional healers and older marabout healers continue longstanding practices of displaying medicines in the open air or in simple repurposed containers. An old traditional healer explained, "Nigériens like local medicines. They want to see, smell, and touch their medicines. Packaging prevents this." In contrast, in the past decade healers of all three medical sectors have increasingly been importing medicines from near and far and thus bringing new choices to Nigériens in Niamey. Every month different new medicines are available. Most of these medicines are packaged and labeled, including some of the traditional medicines, in forms including shrink-wrapped cardboard boxes, tubes and jars for creams, bottles, and blister packs in cardboard boxes. Furthermore, Nigérien traditional and Islamic healers are increasingly packaging their medicines in plastic and paper bags as a strategy to attract patients and increase their profits. "Islamic pharmacists" have emerged as a new category of Islamic healers in Niamey. Finally, informal-sector traditional healers, and to a lesser extent Islamic healers, of Niger are creatively using social media to market their medicines.

Medical mistrust may be more pronounced in Niamey than elsewhere, but some degree of mistrust is inherent in virtually all asymmetrical power relationships between healers and patients. Taking mistrust seriously and paying attention to strategies for overcoming mistrust can reveal much about what is meaningful to people in Niger or to people everywhere in the world. Mistrust is much more than simply a destructive force or the opposite of trust. It can be a practical approach for dealing with ambiguity and it can be productive in the sense that it contributes to medical pluralism, providing multiple therapeutic options for patients and openings for healers to make a living. Finally,

I assert that consideration of the material culture of medicine can generate critical insights on the workings of the mistrust–trust continuum.

Although these various street healers work hard to minimize people's mistrust, this does not mean that it disappears. In fact, mistrust remains prevalent and can flare up in particular health contexts. In the following chapter, I will focus on how the mistrust–trust continuum played out in Niamey during a contemporary public health crisis, the COVID-19 pandemic. I will draw on earlier discussions of the history of the ways that mistrust of biomedicine and mistrust of the government are intertwined. Ultimately, I will argue that the state was unable to overcome the mistrust of Nigériens and explain why.

CHAPTER 6

# Expressing Doubts About COVID-19
# and Fear of Vaccinations in Niger

"Niger is the Land That Covid-19 Forgot," declared a *Wall Street Journal* headline (Faucon 2021). Epidemiologists have been unable to explain why Niger in particular and Africa in general have been impacted far less by COVID-19 than other regions of the world. Furthermore, Niger had the fewest cases of any country in West Africa (R. Idrissa 2021, 38). This is part of the reason Nigériens have their own explanations about the pandemic, as will become clear below. According to state and international monitoring data, as of December 23, 2021, "only" 7,185 confirmed cases and 272 confirmed deaths[1] had been recorded; and as of December 23, 2023, "only" 9,515 confirmed cases and 315 deaths had been recorded in Niger since the onset of the pandemic in a population of about 25 million (Our World in Data 2021, 2023).

Niger avoided a major crisis with the disease itself, and that is critical to how Nigériens think about it. Nigériens may have some resistance as the youngest population in the world with a median age of 15 years, and due to the dry heat of the Sahel, their largely outdoor culture, and possible long-term exposure to earlier variants of the coronavirus (Faucon 2021; R. Idrissa 2021; Sams and Hrynick 2020), but these factors are insufficient to resolve the mystery because other behaviors would seem to make Nigériens particularly vulnerable to the virus. These include densely crowded compounds in Niamey and throughout Niger, very low levels of regular handwashing with soap, the widespread practice of communal dining with shared plates and drinking vessels, and the common sharing of plastic tea kettles of water for ritual ablutions at mosques or wherever people happen to be at prayer times.

This involves the daily touching of lips to the pots as well as breathing into the water that dozens of people use.

While the low incidence of death due to COVID-19 remains largely a mystery, what is clear is that many Nigériens in Niamey had their already precarious lives upended during the initial months of the pandemic, which deepened mistrust of biomedicine and the state. This chapter offers a contemporary—if extreme—example of the complexly contextual nature of the mistrust of biomedicine and biomedical messaging in Niger. As I argued in Chapter 2, biomedicine per se is not mistrusted by Nigériens. Indeed, millions of Nigériens rely on biomedical consultations, pharmaceutical drugs, and vaccines as an important part of their overall therapeutic routines. Vaccine avoidance is highly contextual in Niger. A very high percentage of people in Niamey (85 percent) and Maradi (92 percent) were eager to get meningitis and cholera vaccinations during outbreaks of those diseases in 2021 while most Nigériens were resisting COVID-19 vaccinations, as I noted in Chapter 2. What was and is different about COVID-19? An important part of the answer is that most Nigériens sense that emergency public health campaigns by the state focus on the wrong problems rather than more pressing health concerns.

I did not travel to Niger in 2021 intending to study COVID-19. However, many Nigériens were still talking about the pandemic and thus I altered my plans and seized the opportunity to examine the ways medical mistrust operates during and in the aftermath of a specific public health crisis. I argue that this contemporary example illustrates many of the core themes developed in this book as they unfolded, including the history of medical mistrust; the multidimensional nature of mistrust; the different ways Nigériens experienced COVID-19, influenced by class, gender, religion, and other variables; and the reality that mistrust and trust are contextual and can change over time. In this chapter, more than in previous ones, I emphasize the power of conversation and storytelling in spreading mistrust. Furthermore, to this point, I have not seriously considered "race" in terms of mistrust because Nigériens rarely mentioned it in interviews, focus groups, or everyday conversations.[2] In contrast, many of the narratives about COVID-19 circulating in Niamey express a racial dimension to medical mistrust.

I will focus on analysis of extreme doubts about COVID-19 and mistrust and fear of COVID-19 tests and vaccinations among Nigériens in Niamey, highlighting the ways that these doubts are framed and articulated. I argue that this skepticism can be interpreted through the lens of history as well as contemporary realities and mysteries. For various reasons Nigériens have long mistrusted crisis-framed, Western-influenced public health interventions—such as those associated with HIV-AIDS and polio—imposed by their government, as I discussed in Chapter 3. Nigérien state policies—adhering to WHO guidelines—designed to mitigate the spread of the pandemic led to economic, social, and religious deprivation, and hence deep resentment among most people. Nigériens *may* have had a different perspective on the pandemic and may have been more tolerant of emergency state mandates *if* they had perceived COVID-19 as a serious public health crisis. But the vast majority of Nigériens say that they do not know anyone who contracted the virus or died from it, and data collected by state and international monitors indicates that their perceptions are essentially accurate. The everyday politics of health and the state are what is at stake in Niger. Nigériens widely mistrusted their government long before the COVID-19 pandemic for many reasons, including endemic corruption and the state's inability to provide adequate, affordable health care or defend the country's borders against terrorist attacks. As well-intentioned as the Nigérien government's policies regarding the pandemic may have been, they pushed Nigériens to a tipping point. I suggest that at this historical moment, the Nigérien state has lost what little trust and credibility it had among Nigériens, and that the government would likely find it nearly impossible to mobilize citizens to follow public health mandates and guidelines in the event of a real crisis that might kill many people.[3]

I am particularly interested in unraveling the conclusions that Nigériens are drawing about COVID-19 that are shared through stories and rumors in everyday conversation. I found that 90 percent of Nigériens in Niamey trust one or more of the most commonly circulating narratives. First, COVID-19 is a scam and does not exist. Second, COVID-19 exists but Nigériens are largely immune to it due either to the hot climate of Niger, Islam, or Blackness, or all three working together. Third, COVID-19 is a massive case of blowback from a nefarious Western plot to sterilize and kill Africans that went awry and primarily kills Whites and others. Despite the differences in these narratives, they share the theme that Nigériens have no reason to fear COVID-19. Most Nigériens are aware of these different readings and typically do not see them as contradictory. Furthermore, and by extension, many Nigériens regard COVID-19 tests and vaccinations as sinister strategies to sterilize or kill them. Exploring the stories and rumors that circulated in Niger during the COVID-19 pandemic illustrates the important role that conversation plays both in perpetuating mistrust and as a coping mechanism for living with intersecting precarities, including an uncertain medical environment, crushing poverty that was exacerbated by the pandemic, skepticism regarding most official media news sources, and deep mistrust of the state and global institutions.

## State Policies Regarding COVID-19
## and Their Impacts on Nigériens

In December 2019, the UN and the WHO concluded that Africa would be particularly vulnerable to COVID-19 because of the inadequacies of public health care systems on the continent (R. Idrissa 2021, 7). African governments responded in various ways to Western scientific "truth" regarding COVID-19. Madagascar and Tanzania totally rejected WHO-sanctioned narratives, whereas then-President Mahamadou Issoufou and the Nigérien state completely accepted WHO directives and implemented them as quickly and steadfastly as any country in the world, probably in large part because Niger had closely aligned itself with the West and is highly dependent on foreign aid. The Nigérien government, partnering with the WHO, UNICEF, UNFPA, and MSF, established a Comité Technique National COVID-19 that imposed many public health policies designed to protect its citizens beginning on March 13, 2020, six days before the first case of COVID-19 in the country was confirmed (Sams and Hrynick 2020, 17). These included: (1) travel restrictions including closing all of its borders to noncommercial traffic, closing the country's international airport to most noncommercial traffic, two weeks of quarantine under guard for the few people allowed into the country, and isolating Niamey and prohibiting interurban travel; (2) constructing thousands of public handwashing stations and advising people to avoid handshakes; (3) requiring mask-wearing in public; (4) imposing curfews; (5) limiting the number of passengers in taxis; and (6) closing schools and mosques (or requiring physical distancing in them), and banning gatherings of more than 50 people, including gatherings for naming ceremonies, weddings, burial rites, and prayer in mosques.

These policies and information about COVID-19 were widely disseminated though public service announcements (on radio, television, and billboards) produced by the state and a variety of NGOs. For example, on March 17, 2020, President Mahamadou Issoufou appeared on Tele-Sahel, the Nigérien state television channel, to implore Nigériens to take these policies seriously, explaining: "At this time, there is neither treatment nor vaccine against this virus. The only weapon that exists today is prevention" (R. Idrissa 2021, 7). On May 4, 2020, Labor Minister Mohamed Ben Omar died of COVID-19 (Dogru 2020). Tele-Sahel broadcast his words shortly before his death. "COVID-19 is a reality. It is not a state of mind. It kills. It spreads at the speed of light. We must get a grip on ourselves in order to say, 'stop this virus.' It is through discipline alone that will be the weapon to destroy the virus" (Dogru 2020). By September 2020 when very few Nigériens were contracting the virus or dying from it, most of these COVID-19 restrictions were abandoned or only sporadically and situationally enforced, but they left economic misery in their wake and contributed to increasing mistrust of the government and of the coronavirus itself. Later, in early 2021, prominent politicians were shown receiving COVID-19 vaccinations on television. Many Nigériens doubted the veracity of these televised images due to high levels of mistrust in the government (R. Idrissa 2021, 43).

The ways that people initially responded to these public health measures were partly based on socioeconomic class. Political scientist Rahmane Idrissa (2021, 43) argues that the Nigérien "public responded in variable ways, in accordance with the social milieu, the economic activity, and the type of measure." Mistrust of the government is expressed differently by class or social milieu. The Francophone or "modern" class, who make up about 10 percent of Nigériens, focuses its mistrust on perceptions of endemic corruption; "If most Francophones believe the Covid-19 exists and is dangerous, many imagine nonetheless that the government is inflating its impact in Niger in order to obtain more aid money, which—it is assumed—will be misappropriated" (R. Idrissa 2021, 43). The rest of Nigériens, the "popular" classes, center their mistrust on the cultural and especially religious policies of the state. In short, Nigériens mistrusted the state and policies for different reasons based on different class positions and social identities.

During the first weeks of the crisis, most people in Niamey reluctantly accepted most of these measures as necessary for protecting public health, though some Francophones applauded government COVID policies and most other Nigériens were very skeptical. It did not take long for particular "collective ways of questioning these response measures" (Sams et al. 2021, 5) to emerge. As early as April 2020, many Nigériens began not only to ignore these mandates but also to demonstrate publicly against them—especially the closure of mosques— including blocking intersections with burning cars and tires, attacking police stations, and burning a school (AFP 2020; Ben Ahmed 2020; R. Idrissa 2021, 19).

These collective protests and widespread frustration and anger were due in part to the immediate detrimental impact of state policies on Nigériens. For decades, if not centuries, many Nigériens have relied on transnational migration during eight-month-long dry seasons for finding work, and hence the border closures meant crippling loss of income for thousands of people. Many other Nigériens regularly travel abroad and within the country for business and for family visits, and travel restrictions led to financial and personal hardship. An angry and disappointed 60-year-old Fulani man explained, "Due to restrictions I was not able to travel home to Maradi for my father's funeral. This is wrong! I do not know a single person who has COVID-19."

Public health policies designed to slow the spread of COVID-19 exacerbated economic deprivation in Niger. Some people could not go to work, fewer goods were available in markets due to border closures, and night markets—an important part of the informal retail sector in Niamey—were closed because of curfews. According to World Bank estimates, "The number of people in extreme poverty . . . increased by 400,000 as a result of Covid-19 restrictions in 2020" (Faucon 2021). In 2020, there was "a 176% increase in the number of people struggling to meet basic food and other needs" (Sams and Hrynick 2020, 17). In a survey of 3,411 women in Niger from December 2020 to April 2021, 28 percent reported a partial loss of household income and 9 percent reported a total loss of household income (PMA 2021, 2). In a survey of 1,076 women in Niger over the same period, 40 percent reported a partial loss of personal income and 16 percent reported a total loss of personal income (PMA 2021, 2).

Nigériens were also frustrated by directives regarding hygiene and physical contact, some of which went against important cultural practices. Through my long-term research on the economic, cultural, and symbolic dimensions of water in Niamey as well as observations and conversations for decades, I learned that most poor Nigériens think daily ritual ablutions before their five daily Muslim prayers purify and cleanse them and that soap is unnecessary (Keough and Youngstedt 2019, 36, Youngstedt 2013, 58). Most Nigériens in Niamey were thus indifferent to directives to wash hands regularly with soap and water but were willing to do so if soap and water or hand sanitizers were offered free of charge at public places, according to my interviews and conversations. My interlocutors indicated that most poor men in public spaces such as street corner conversation groups, markets, and mosques ignored public health suggestions to avoid handshakes because they are an important part of daily greetings among Nigérien men. Handshaking among men in public spaces was as common when I arrived in July 2021 as it had been before the pandemic began. Middle-class and wealthy men—especially when they were required to do so by government and NGO offices and hotels—washed their hands regularly with soap or sanitizer, substituted fist bumps or elbow bumps for traditional handshakes or avoided touching, and wore masks—again revealing that class differences sometimes led to different perceptions and behaviors.

People in Niamey, especially poor men of Hausa, Zarma-Songhay, and Mawri ethnicity working or socializing outdoors, grew weary of wearing masks. (Men of these groups do not typically cover their faces.). Middle-class men did as well. For example, a middle-aged male aid worker who was having trouble getting his mask to fit properly outside a meeting at the Ministry of Public Health joked, "Masks do not got well with Blacks, but with Whites, oh!, masks go well with Whites" (Squibb 2022). Most residents of Niamey use the French term *bavette* (bib)—and sometimes *masque*—because local languages lack a word for "mask." (There are no masked dance cultures in Niger, unlike in many places closer to the coast in West Africa.) For example, some Hausa use the clunky expression *abin rufe fuska* (a thing that covers the face). However, by the time I arrived in Niamey in July 2021, many people were using the Hausa term *tukunkumi*. This word traditionally refers to muzzles—the type used particularly on ornery camels who would otherwise bite people. In my interpretation, using this term was not merely about trying to find a local word for mask, but reveals intense displeasure about wearing them. As one of my interlocuters who refused to wear a face mask put it, "We are not camels, we are people!" Nigérien men's perspectives on masks varied by ethnicity. Tuareg men, and to some extent Fulani men, customarily cover their faces, and thus pandemic mandates regarding wearing masks did not bother them (Rasmussen 2023, 140). Similarly, women of all ethnic groups in Niamey were increasingly accustomed to wearing veils covering their noses and mouths before the pandemic began due to rising Islamic conservatism. None of the women with whom I spoke complained about wearing masks. Nigérien women rarely use handshakes in their greetings, and almost never shake hands with men. Clearly in Niger there are gendered and ethnic dimensions to norms of physical contact and masking. State policies on physical distancing and masking annoyed many Hausa, Zarma-Songhay, and Mawri men but had little impact on the lives of women and Tuareg and Fulani men.

Many Nigériens in Niamey were confused and alarmed by curfews given that historically curfews have been imposed in Niamey only during coups d'état, and were not during previous large-scale epidemics such as meningitis outbreaks. People of Niamey enjoy going out at night to socialize with family and friends and to shop at night markets when it is relatively cool. This also cut off incomes for traders and restaurateurs, some of whom do most of their business at night. Nigériens would probably oppose COVID-19 curfews regardless of the season, but the fact that they were initially imposed during April and May of 2020—the two hottest months of the year in the Sahel—angered many people.

Niamey residents were also frustrated by the massive disruptions to transportation that these public health initiatives caused. Unlike most large West African cities, Niamey lacks public transportation. Thousands of private four-passenger taxis and 17-passenger *faba* (minibuses in Zarma) serve this role. Long before COVID-19 taxi and *faba* drivers' profit margin was razor-thin because of the high cost of gasoline and long-imposed restrictions on fares. Physical distancing mandates that limited taxis to two passengers at a time put many taxi drivers in debt or out of business altogether (R. Idrissa 2021, 31–34; Faucon 2021). Many bush taxi drivers and their assistants who provide intercity transportation in minibuses suffered too because of prohibitions on intercity travel. Rahmane Idrissa (2021, 34) emphasized the ripple effect of this problem: "The social and economic consequences of the crisis extend beyond the misery of transportation workers. In most cases, these workers are breadwinners for their family . . . The freezing of minibus stations wrecked the street trading of small retailers, coaxers, snack vendors, [mechanics], that flourished around them." The policy also frustrated passengers because their trips were delayed, and drivers were forced to drive a harder bargain than before the restrictions were imposed.

No policy generated more resistance and protest than the prohibition on gatherings of 50 or more people, particularly for Muslim prayers and rites of passage. Rahmane Idrissa (2021, 44) drew the same conclusion, and highlights how this policy fueled mistrust of the government, COVID-19, and the West: "The government's decision to prohibit large religious gatherings and close mosques to Friday prayers turned skepticism into outrage. Soon, stories propagated from northern Nigeria gave structure and focus to the outrage by claiming that Covid-19 was an invention of the West, which intended to destroy Islam by undermining the practice of religion." Many of my interviewees also expressed anger about the disruption of communal prayer. One middle-aged Hausa man expressed his anger with insults, "Our leaders are Jews and pagans, they do not care about Islam, and they do not pray." His

Zarma friend offered a broader critique regarding the closing of mosques: "Islam is under assault around the world. For two years in a row Saudi Arabia has prevented foreigners traveling to Mecca for the Muslim pilgrimage, proving the Saudi Arabia is a puppet of Europe and the U.S. My father never received a refund for the ticket he bought for the pilgrimage last year. We must be allowed to pray in our mosques."

Further concern about how government policies were interfering with religious practice were associated with the state requirement that people who had died of COVID-19 be buried by health officials and firefighters. Many Nigériens were outraged. An old Tuareg man's objections were typical of this sentiment: "This upset our long tradition whereby families are responsible for completing proper Islamic burial rites." Many Nigériens also objected to physical distancing policies that were required in some mosques that were allowed to remain open or were reopened later when policies were loosened. A 25-year-old Fulani man explained, "We are expected to pray close together. If we are separated due to COVID-19 policies, Satan can sneak into the spaces between us and trick us." Many Nigériens simply ignored the policy on gatherings (C. Idrissa 2021, Nowak 2021). Security agents of the state were mobilized to patrol the streets of Niamey to identify and arrest recalcitrant people.

Most West African countries closed mosques and churches in the initial weeks and months of the pandemic. However, churches in Niger were allowed to remain open, and this added to the sense among some Nigériens that Islam was under siege and to even more mistrust of the government.[4] Unlike most countries in the region, authorities in Niger permitted markets to remain open, except for night markets, during the time curfew was being enforced, as mentioned earlier. Most Nigériens were very pleased with this decision. However, many of my interlocuters emphasized the contradiction in prohibiting mosque gatherings while allowing markets to remain open. A young Zarma man explained his take on the conflicting policies: "It makes no sense. You know how crowded our markets are. If these restrictions were really about protecting public health, both markets and mosques would be closed. I think the government is against Islam. Plus, they do not understand that many of us think it is more important to have mosques open than markets."

In contrast, a minority of people used the Hausa proverb *mutuwar wani rai wani* (the death of one is the life of another) to describe the economic opportunities that opened to some Nigériens as a result of COVID-19 and state policies in the context of precarity. These opportunities were narrow considering all the economic disruption and hardship faced by so many, but on a small scale local tailors briefly appreciated the extra work making masks and so did hundreds of children who were employed to sell them on the street (Nowak 2021). Entrepreneurs capitalized on the expanded market for hand sanitizers and liquid soap. Blacksmiths and carpenters profited from the construction of handwashing stations. Many tailors, children, entrepreneurs, and craftsmen expressed disappointment when the market for masks, more soap than usual, and handwashing stations largely evaporated around September 2020 (Nowak 2021).

The government of Niger offered some "compensatory measures" as part of its overall COVID policy (R. Idrissa 2021, 12–13). These included a variety of economic and fiscal measures such as suspending collection of overdue taxes and waiving taxes on certain products, and a range of social support measures such as "a waiving of household water and electricity bills for the months of April and May . . . adoption of a price ceiling for certain products (grain and household necessities) . . . [and] early release of 1,540 prisoners (older, juvenile, women, ill)" (R. Idrissa 2021, 13). These policies mitigated financial hardship for a minority of Nigériens. However, they were fundamentally flawed in that the people who needed assistance the most were largely excluded from access to it. Only people and businesses in the formal sector—less than 10 percent—could access the economic and fiscal benefits. Waiving of electricity and water bills did nothing to help millions of Nigériens who are too poor to live "on the grid" and instead rely on kerosene lanterns and pay for informal-sector water delivery or well water (Keough and Young-stedt 2019). In sum, these public health policies only further contributed to people's views—especially among the poor—that the state was not genuinely interested in their health and well-being.

These policies may have helped mitigate the spread of the virus, but they came with a high cost. Mohamed Bazoum, while he was the interior minister in 2020—he became the president in 2021—concluded that, "We killed a fly with a hammer . . . the coronavirus arrived but it never prospered" (Faucon 2021). By this he meant that Niger's policies were far stricter than they needed to be. Dr. Amadou Foumakoye Gado, head of COVID-19 services at Niamey's Lamordé Reference Hospital, indicated in a July 2021 interview that "In the last month, we have not had a single patient in intensive care. We have reallocated respirators to other sectors of the hospital that have more need of them" (Faucon 2021).

In Niger as elsewhere in Africa, "Preemptive government measures to contain viral spread compounded preexisting uncertainties in health, livelihoods, and citizen-state relations" (MacGregor et al. 2021, 1). *Indeed, state COVID-19 policies had a far greater negative impact than the virus itself on the vast majority of Nigériens.* (MacGregor et al. 2021, 1) suggest that "The notion of 'intersecting precarities' to encapsulate this reality of COVID-19 manifesting amidst already precarious lives and a paucity of state welfare, prompting people to take individual and collective action to negotiate the effects of public health restrictions." As noted earlier, in April 2020 and in the following months Nigériens began ignoring public health mandates and publicly demonstrated against what many perceived to be "drastic measures" (C. Idrissa 2020) to combat the pandemic. The state arrested "anyone who spoke publicly against the campaign to fight the pandemic" including medical doctors and "vocal clerics it considered threats to the success of the pandemic policy" (R. Idrissa 2021, 19). Given the respect that Nigériens have for Muslim leaders, "Throngs of supporters took to the streets, clamouring for the release of 'our cleric,' attacking police stations, and in Mirriah . . . burning down a school, seen as a fount of the impious Western culture of the government" (R. Idrissa 2021, 19).

Most Nigériens mistrusted the state and large-scale biomedical interventions long before COVID-19, as highlighted in earlier chapters. The government's violent suppression of demonstrations and "use of COVID-19 as justification for recent political repression" (Sams and Hrynick 2020, 18), further fueled mistrust of the state and biomedicine. Furthermore, there is not much state welfare in Niger, where the government treats most people as the population rather than as citizens. Health care in Niger is centered on personal social relations and networks of family, friends, Muslim scholars, herbalists, and street vendors. In sum, the example of COVID-19 shows mistrust is not static and can fluctuate depending on circumstance. In this case, a range of state policies exacerbated existing challenges and laid bare the state's inability or disinterest in caring for its citizens.

By July 2021, 16 months into the pandemic, when I arrived after a two-year absence, most of these public health policies had long been abandoned or were no longer being enforced. About one in 50 people were wearing face masks and handwashing stations had disappeared. Notable exceptions included some state and NGO offices as well as luxury hotels that required face masks, especially at large events, and where many people were substituting fist-bumps for traditional handshakes or avoiding physical contact altogether.

Markets, mosques, and taxis were densely crowded with people. I was told repeatedly that COVID-19 is not real, or if it is, Nigériens are immune to it for various reasons. Coming from the U.S. where I had been primarily isolated at home and forced to teach online, assiduously masked and observing physical distancing policies when I occasionally ventured out, I felt as though I was visiting a parallel universe. Nigérien friends, contacts, and people that I met listened to my stories of COVID-19 in the U.S. and regularly asked me about it before, during, and after my visit, but I felt that they were doing so just to be polite. A few days into my visit, I went to see my old friend Elhadji Lamine, owner of a construction supply business, at his office. He asked with a broad grin, "You are not afraid to shake hands, are you?" Given that I was fully vaccinated, I responded, "No," and we shook hands, shared laughter about it, and spent an hour together catching up about our families and life. He was not concerned about shaking hands but knew I might be hesitant. Alternatively, he may have been applying the logic of Nigérien medical mistrust to me. That is, he may have acknowledged that I might not trust the U.S. government's assessment regarding the risks of COVID-19. After all, I was not wearing a mask and I had traveled thousands of miles to be there.

Finally, I argue that since so few Nigériens believe in the existence of, or threat posed by, COVID-19 there is no market for COVID-19 medicines in Niamey. Despite an Islamic pharmacist's attempt to sell me medicine to treat COVID-19 as I discussed in Chapter 3, I neither encountered nor heard news of any Nigérien healers—traditional, Islamic, or biomedical—who claimed to have COVID-19-specific medicine. In contrast, many purported COVID cures have emerged around the world, such as "Covid Cure (1)" by the Abdelleh brothers in Ghana (Atuire et al. 2021), elephant dung in Namibia (Ogala 2021, 305), the herbal tonic "Covid Organics" in Madagascar (Ogala 2021, 310), and U.S. President Trump's hydroxychloroquine, bleach injections, and bright lights treatments.

## Mistrust and Rumors Regarding COVID-19 in Niger

In their study of migrant gold miners in Suriname and French Guiana, Heemskerk et al. (2022) found that "In a life full of risks, COVID-19 makes little difference." The gold miners there faced "intersecting precarities" (MacGregor et al. 2021, 1) long before COVID-19 in the form of malaria, snakes, corrupt police, and dangerous working conditions. Given this reality they expressed little concern about COVID-19, seeing it as just another risk and not the most dangerous one in their lives. They trusted home remedies and over-the-counter medicines for treating COVID-19, and sought biomedical attention in only the most extreme cases. Living in the world's least developed country, many Nigériens live with "intersecting precarities" such as poverty, violence, climate change, and government instability and express a similar nonchalant attitude about the pandemic. Nigériens who suspect that they have COVID-19 also prefer traditional medicine and "over the counter" pharmaceuticals purchased from street vendors to seeking treatment in clinics and hospitals. However, in contrast with the South American miners studied by Heemskerk et al. (2022), many Nigériens in Niamey have come to question the very existence of COVID-19, think they are protected from it if it does exist, or are convinced that it was deliberately manufactured in a genocidal plot against Africans and Muslims. These perspectives illustrate prevailing medical mistrust as well as mistrust of global health institutions and the state among Nigériens.

Nigériens who acknowledge the global reality of COVID-19 have their own ideas about how climate, race, and religion have protected them. Most of the people I interviewed and spoke with point to the hot, arid climate of Niger as protective. As one 35-year-old man put it, "COVID-19 does not survive in very hot temperatures, and Niger is very hot. Thus, it is the sun that hinders the advance of COVID-19." Traditionally sedentary ethnic groups of southern Niger such as the Hausa, Zarma-Songhay, and Mawri tend to be darker-completed than the traditionally nomadic ethnic groups of northern Niger such as Tuareg, Fulani, and Arab. Some Nigériens refer to the former as Blacks and the latter as Whites. Many Black Nigériens expressed the belief that the virus is a White people's problem, and that Black Africans have natural immunity due to their Blackness. A "Black" Hausa man commented on this idea, "Does the coronavirus exist? No. It is just a simple cold that we already know. Historically, Whites, Arabs, Fulani, and Tuareg cannot handle colds and die quickly from them." Many more ominous rumors and stories involving racial themes circulated in Niamey, such as one told by a 50-year-old Hausa man: "Whites created COVID-19 to kill Blacks, but somehow their plan backfired, and it only kills Whites."

Many Nigériens think that Islam keeps the safe from COVID-19. Rahmane Idrissa (2021, 18), recognizing the enormous influence of Muslim leaders in Niger, noted that "In mid-March [2020], a prominent Izala leader, Mallam Sani Yahaya Jingir, made a fiery sermon on Izala TV in which he described 'corona' as a Western plot against Muslims and later also said that the disease was not real. Videos of crowds of his supporters chanting that 'corona is not real' went viral on WhatsApp and widely circulated in Niger." Cheiffou Idrissa (2021) similarly observed that most imams—the most respected leaders in Niger—preached that COVID-19 does not exist or is not a threat to Nigériens and did nothing to encourage their congregations to follow public health guidelines. Like some other Islamic scholars, Elhadji Ousseini preached to his congregation that "COVID-19 is divine punishment that was already planned by Allah. When communities are perverted, misfortune will always befall them." He explained that since Muslim communities are not perverted, they have no reason to fear COVID-19. Indeed, many Nigériens claim that Allah is safeguarding them because they are Muslims. A 45-year-old Tuareg man's comments were typical among the people I interviewed: "People have more fear of God than of COVID-19. Nothing happens without his will, and he has chosen to protect us." However, it is important to remember that Islam in Niger is not monolithic. Some prominent clerics recognized the reality of COVID-19 and its potential danger, used Islamic principles regarding the sacredness of life to encourage people to adhere to state guidelines, and pointed out that Saudi Arabia had also closed its mosques (R. Idrissa 2021, 20). Many people mentioned that the interaction of climate, race, and religion keep Nigériens safe from COVID-19.

By July 2021—and probably much earlier—few Nigériens in Niamey feared COVID-19 because 90 percent thought it was nothing new or that they enjoyed multidimensional protection against it. The most common comment by far that was made in interviews and conversations was: "We are used to runny noses and influenza, we have them all the time, this is no different." A 40-year-man Fulani man who works as a driver for a humanitarian NGO and is aware of COVID-19 precautions explained, "When you read the list of symptoms for COVID, I must have had COVID four times in the last year" (Squibb 2022)— illustrating how often people are sick with fevers, coughs, sore throats, etc. A young Hausa woman expressed confusion in a way that was representative of many of the people with whom I spoke: "Sometimes you can have all of the so-called symptoms and test negative for COVID-19, and other times you can have none of the symptoms and test positive for COVID-19. I think it is a scam. I do not think COVID-19 exists." Nigériens with colds and suspected COVID-19 typically self-medicate with home botanical remedies or pharmaceutical drugs purchased from mobile street vendors. Indeed, the most common treatment used by Nigériens to treat COVID-19 is the same treatment used for colds—hot water with lemon, ginger, honey, and sometimes garlic. A wide range of pharmaceutical cold medicines, such as paracetamol and Kold Time, were also popular for treating coronavirus symptoms.

Some Nigériens shifted their perspectives over time, primarily from one of some initial fear to just ignoring the whole pandemic as much as possible. In contrast, Idrissa, a 55-year-old humanitarian aid worker, said to me in person in July 2021, "Ninety-five percent of Nigériens do not believe that COVID-19 exists, and I am one of them," but by late December 2021, he informed me via email that, "For sure, COVID-19 has seriously returned to Niger because of the cold, wind, and dust." Many Nigériens with whom I spoke noticed spikes in cases in December 2020–January 2021, December 2021–January 2022, and December 2022–January 2023, that were documented by international monitors (Our World in Data 2023). This coincides with the cold season in Niger when harmattan winds kick up dust that leads to colds, respiratory ailments, and meningitis epidemics—all of which have symptoms like those of COVID-19.

Nigérien rumors about COVID-19 emerged against a backdrop of increasing difficulty telling a fake—be it a news story, cell phone, or medical treatment—from the real in Niger. Kingori (2021, 339) observes that "In recent years, and especially during the Covid-19 pandemic, there has been mounting concern expressed in public and scholarly domains about fakes in African spaces," including political corruption, false narratives, reproductions of material culture, counterfeit medicines, and fake diseases. However, Africa is not unique regarding concerns about fake news and misinformation. These are issues all over the world that are integral to the politics of health and state. On a global scale in the first year of the pandemic, the "WHO warned against the scourge of 'infodemics' or the overabundance of false stories making it difficult for people to make sense of the Covid-19 pandemic" (Ogala 2021, 305). Ogala (2021, 307–308) argues that today's world is defined by a "complex and layered contestation over who gets to define the truth and the fake, and under what terms." Kingori (2021, 245) argues that "The existence of or argument for 'fake news' depends on the idea that there is a real authentic, true news that we should believe and yet Africans have had a long history of being the recipients of false accounts from the Global North." In terms of the medical science and technology of COVID-19, "Legitimacy and authenticity are determined by fragile and arbitrary systems constructed and governed by institutions in the global North" (Kingori 2021, 250). Furthermore, as

Ogala (2021) emphasizes, there is enduring—though misplaced—concern that Africans are particularly susceptible to false narratives. Despite the lack of evidence to support it, this Eurocentric position endures due to continuing racist ideas about the mental inferiority of Africans that fails to take account of historical, political, economic, and socioeconomic context. The circulation of rumors and stories in Niamey regarding White conspiracies to decimate Black Africans through COVID-19 itself or through vaccinations to counteract it must be read in the historical context of past Western-led health initiatives, such as family planning and mass vaccination campaigns that sterilized, harmed, or killed Nigériens and other Africans (Archibong and Annan 2001; Fatunde and Familusi 2001; Masquelier 2012; May 2017; Renne 2010).

Doubt, rumors, and conspiracy theories regarding COVID-19 and vaccinations have been circulating since the onset of the pandemic and continue to circulate globally. Nigériens are aware of them through a wide range of sources and particularly Radio France Internationale (RFI) reporting that has long been their most popular source of global news. Stewart and Strathern (2003) emphasize that rumors flourish in situations involving uncertainty and often connect the local to the global. Different people in particular places have different reasons for questioning the reality of the virus and the purpose of vaccines. For example, suspicions of falseness or fraud in one area—for example, believing that COVID-19 is a lie or a deliberate White conspiracy to attack Black bodies as many Nigériens do—are related to suspicions in others, such as the widespread belief that the Nigérien state is merely a puppet of France. In the politics of state and health, the more the state is mistrusted, the more its health policies and mandates are questioned or dismissed altogether. Most Nigériens began to doubt Western scientific facts about COVID-19 within weeks or months of the onset of the pandemic. Horror stories of experiments on children, sterilization, and death "help construct and legitimise a racialised narrative of suspicion around which local populations can easily be mobilised" (Ogala 2021, 308–309).

The sterilization stories currently circulating in Niamey are nuanced in particular ways while echoing a theme expressed by Africans and people of African descent worldwide for centuries. Rekia, a 50-year-old Mawri woman, put the concerns of Nigériens into historical context: "France and other foreign countries have always tried to reduce our population through slavery and forced labor and now through trickery like family planning, vaccines, and Corona. We think Corona and the vaccine were designed to sterilize us and thus weaken us so they can take more of our resources." In her analysis of rumors told by African Americans in the U.S. about White plots to sterilize and kill them with secret ingredients in food products, Turner (1993, 3) argues that "Organized anti-black conspiracies threaten the communal well-being and, in particular, the individual bodies of blacks," and emphasizes the "pervasiveness of metaphors linking the fate of the black race to the fates of black bodies, metaphors in use since the very first contact between whites and blacks." Kaler (2009, 1711) found that skepticism among Africans about public health interventions is expressed through rumors, and that "One recurrent theme [found in more than 30 cases scattered across the continent] in such rumours is the centrality of reproductive bodies (both male and female); and the perception that these bodies are rendered sterile by toxic compounds given under the guise of improving health." The sterility theme also bears some similarities with a genre of stories about bloodsucking shared in colonial East and Central Africa (White 2000) in which Africans were terrorized by White occupiers who pretended to help them.

Following historian Luise White's perspective in *Speaking with Vampires*, I argue that it is important to take rumors seriously, not simply rumors per se but rather the "world that rumor and gossip reveals" (2000, 5). Nigérien stories about lethal racist and Islamophobic plots are credible and worth repeating even by those who do not necessarily fully believe them because they seem plausible and reasonable in a context of extreme mistrust of international institutions, France, the Nigérien government, and crisis-framed public health messaging and policies. These rumors should not be dismissed as superstitions or misunderstandings. Stories and rumors are "concrete and frequently analytical expressions of Africans' experiences" (White 2021, 320). Like similar stories told by other Africans, Nigérien stories about COVID-19 and vaccinations "might be exaggerated, they might be metaphorical . . . but as a description of [global racial neocolonial capitalist inequality] they are not wrong" (White 2021, 321). Furthermore, they coexist with official stories. The speed of storytelling disrupts the true–false binary.

Nigérien voices regarding COVID-19 "subvert the power structures in place which create and then legitimise 'the real' and 'the authentic'" (Kingori 2021, 249). Despite global structures of exclusion and domination, Nigériens are claiming space to construct an "alternative regime of truth" (Ogala 2021, 310) and meaning. Nigérien rumors and "'fake news' speaks to and responds to exclusion" (Kingori 2021, 244), serving as "weapons of the weak" (Scott

1985). Nigériens do not gain any "practical" or economic advantages by denying global biomedical truths about the pandemic and resisting vaccination,
and they might be endangering themselves if a new particularly virulent strain
of the virus emerges. However, their rumors and stories enable them to feel a
sense of pride and agency in the face of intersecting precarities, global racial
capitalism, Islamophobia, and institutions and states that they have good reason to mistrust. Furthermore, the plausibility of Nigérien rumors denying the
danger of COVID-19 is enhanced by the fact that so few Nigériens have died
from it, but most Nigériens in Niamey have suffered in one way or another
from state health policies and mandates.

### Fear of Testing and Vaccinations in Niamey

Most Nigériens think that COVID-19 testing and vaccines are unnecessary
since they do not perceive coronavirus as a threat to their health. Many are
also mistrustful and fearful of these interventions on the grounds that they
are part of a master scheme to sterilize or kill them. Beginning with testing, aid worker Eliza Squibb (2022) offered analysis based on her experience
in Niamey in early 2021 that matches my observations: "In general, when
people have COVID-19 symptoms, they are strongly reluctant to get tested
because they do not know what the government would do if they tested positive. They fear they would be forced to go quarantine somewhere and lose
their freedom. They prefer not to know or disclose if they have COVID-19.
People played down their symptoms and did not directly say that they had
COVID. Instead, they say, 'I have malaria and a cough,' a Nigérien code for 'I
have COVID.'" The reasons why Nigériens are not getting tested are new—the
state is feared more than the coronavirus—but they may also illustrate an attitude identified by Last (1992) who found "that not-knowing and not-caring-
to-know are genuine attitudes of mind and that they are very important to
the [Hausa] medical culture" (Last 1992, 394). In his long-term research, Last
observed that many Hausa prefer a lack of information about certain illnesses
because not knowing can be better than knowing in some circumstances. In
the case of COVID-19, Nigériens fear that the tests themselves may be dangerous and that the potential consequences of testing positive include forced
detention and vaccinations with a sterilizing agent.

Many of the small minority of Nigériens who were interested in getting
tested for COVID-19 were unsure of where to go and how much it would cost,

even though free rapid tests have been available at the Centre de Recherche Médicale et Sanitaire (CERMES) operated by the Ministère da la Santé Publique. A Nigérien project manager "was surprised that the rapid testing was free and open to Nigériens in addition to foreign aid workers, so probably no one knew about it" (Squibb 2022). The high cost of PCR tests contributed to the sense that testing was simply a money-grabbing scam. PCR tests cost 5,000 CFA as a prerequisite for interurban highway travel in Niger and 25,000 CFA for air travel, or about 10 and 50 times the daily per capita income in Niger, respectively.

Beginning in March 2021, the Ministère da la Santé Publique initiated a "mass campaign of vaccination" against COVID-19, initially with vaccines donated by China and later using ones donated by the U.S. However, very few Nigériens initially opted to accept vaccines, even though—or in some ways *because*—they are offered free of charge. Because there was such low demand in the country, on May 30, 2021, Niger "loaned" Côte d'Ivoire 100,000 doses of the AstraZeneca COVID-19 vaccine (Ouestafnews 2021). Ouestafnews (2021) reported that technically this was a loan, but their interpretation is that it is highly unlikely that Niger will ask Côte d'Ivoire for the same number of vaccines in the future, and hence the use of the word *prêt* (loan) in quotes in their headline. By November 28, 2021, 971,636 doses had been administered in Niger and 469,051 Nigériens were fully vaccinated (Our World in Data 2021). Thus, only 2 percent of Nigériens were fully vaccinated by late 2021. These numbers gradually rose in the following 19 months. After more than three years of the pandemic, as of July 30, 2023, 23.8 percent of Nigériens had received at least one dose of the COVID-19 vaccine (Our World in Data 2023).

The relatively small number of officially reported cases of COVID-19 and deaths attributed to it may also contribute to refusals to accept vaccinations. However, this alone is insufficient as an explanation for the widespread fear of COVID-19 vaccinations. For example, in 2021, a story circulated that France was testing COVID-19 vaccines on children in the Koubia neighborhood of Niamey and perhaps others. This rumor provoked immediate action. One witness saw "women run to pick up their children from school" to remove them from harm's way. Although the "news" was false and the rumor was short-lived, the fact that it was told, circulated, and that some people believed it and took direct action on it illustrates a "racialised narrative of suspicion" (Ogala 2021, 309) that cuts across ideas about the pandemic, state and global responses, testing, and vaccinations.

The fear of testing and vaccinations is not occurring in a historical vacuum. Nigériens have long been highly mistrustful of Western-generated, crisis-framed approaches to public health, especially in situations that are not perceived as a crisis, and they do not perceive that COVID-19 is one. Furthermore, millions of Nigériens who are refusing COVID-19 vaccines have never received any vaccine, and millions more have only had one or two vaccines when they were infants or children and had no say in the matter. Finally, many of the people I spoke with in July 2021—and not just the older ones— referred to stories of counterfeit meningitis vaccines administered in Niger in the 1990s that had allegedly killed thousands of children as well as the vaccination catastrophe in nearby Kano, Nigeria, in 1996. In that episode, Pfizer, deploying an experimental meningitis vaccine, Trovan, "selected a sample of 200 children between 3 months and 18 years old to participate. A month later, 11 of the children that had participated were dead. Additionally, numerous parents of children involved in the trials reported disabilities among their children, including paralysis and liver failure" (Archibong and Annan 2021).

Nigériens express their reluctance to accept vaccinations in a variety of terms. I was repeatedly told that vaccinations were designed to sterilize or kill African Muslims—part of an ongoing plot that began with family planning and polio and other vaccination campaigns. A middle-aged Hausa man described a sinister motive: "The Whites want to robotize [control] us. They seek all means and methods to reduce the number of Africans." A middle-aged Zarma woman explained her fear of COVID-19 vaccinations, "There is no such thing as a free lunch. There must be a catch." A young Zarma woman expressed her reticence about COVID-19 vaccinations: "Must we get vaccinated? No, Allah will protect me. I will not get one unless the authorities render it obligatory. The same is true in Europe where some people are refusing to get vaccinated." A Chadian musician who resides in Niamey and regularly travels to France complained, "Europe will let us back in once they have sold us their vaccine" (Squibb 2021). He believes that big pharmaceutical companies control the world and have created COVID-19 vaccines solely to generate profits. A young Hausa man explained: "I am healthy and so I have not gone to get a shot. A certain friend of mine was said to have COVID-19. A doctor gave him medicine and told him to drink it. He did not drink it and then the doctors took him to a control center, and the control center said that he was healed [free of COVID-19] and released him. I repeat, he did not drink the medicine that they gave him." His story addresses many common themes: doubt about the reality of the virus, mistrust of biomedicine, and fear of the state and detention. Furthermore, several participants in my research indicated that negative PCR test results and vaccination cards can be obtained through bribery or through an underground market for about 10,000 CFA each.

Refusing testing and vaccinations and the vaccine campaign itself have had negative impacts for public health in Niger that extend beyond the COVID-19 pandemic because "Intense resource mobilization to fight the Covid-19 outbreak threatened operation and progress in the larger health-care system" (R. Idridssa 2021, 41). According to Sams and Hrynick (2020, 20), "In the context of COVID -19, there is evidence that people may avoid health facilities and basic care for fear of infection with the virus, or a positive COVID-19 test that would lead to isolation and forced hospitalization," as highlighted earlier. A few examples illustrate this point. Many people who visited CSI community clinics did not receive the services they sought as a result of a 50 percent reduction in staff (and staff working alternate days) due to physical distancing policies (Squibb 2022). From December 2020 to April 2021, 18 percent of women were unsuccessful in securing general health consultations, and there was a 38 percent decline in the number of women seeking family planning services (PMA 2021)—further fueling the feeling that the government was neglecting them. Furthermore, as Sams and Hrynick (2020, 14) point out, "Recent polio outbreaks in 2020 have also been linked to the suspension of [polio] vaccination campaigns due to COVID-19" and the emphasis on COVID-19 vaccination efforts. Finally, Squibb (2022) observed that "Public health workers must run monthly campaigns to try to get their numbers up to meet donor standards when they are struggling so much to get people to accept Covid vaccinations and would much rather focus on more urgent health campaigns."

In sum, Nigériens' hesitancy to accept COVID-19 tests and vaccinations is clearly linked to their sense that they are not threatened by COVID-19. Even many of those who acknowledge the existence of COVID-19 are reluctant to get tested and vaccinated for various reasons. Some fear that they are a devious ploy to sterilize them. Others are content to rely on faith. Still others think tests and vaccines are just a money-making scam by Big Pharma. Finally, the Nigérien state's emphasis on COVID-19 vaccinations was detrimental to its overall delivery of public health services, contributing to further mistrust of the government.

## Conclusion

Nigérien state policies that followed Western directives were far more disruptive in terms of the economy, social life, and religious practice than COVID-19 itself, exacerbating the vulnerability of and angering Nigériens. Nigériens resisted state and global directives by ignoring and protesting against them, and by creating and circulating narratives that challenge their exclusion from global decision-making. These stories are often racialized and point to a failed White conspiracy to attack Black bodies through either the virus or vaccines or both. Other stories emphasize attacks on Islamic practice. These narratives express the strength and agency of Black Muslims living in the Sahel in the context of global racial neocolonial capitalist inequality.

In this chapter, I have attempted to elucidate the historical and cultural logics that have led Nigériens in Niamey draw particular conclusions about COVID-19. Nigérien perspectives on COVID-19 must be read in the context of pervasive mistrust of the state, which was exacerbated by its pandemic response, the history of mistrust of emergency health measures based on coercion rather than persuasion, the nebulous nature of COVID symptoms, and the low number of cases. Most Nigériens saw no good reason to think that COVID-19 threatened them or to trust the entities that told them that they must be protected from it. The association of COVID-19 with sterility reveals the intensity of Nigérien thoughts and feeling on the matter, because infertility is Nigériens' greatest health concern as it brings shame and social death (Cooper 2019; Moussa 2023).

In the conclusion, I will extend this analysis by comparing medical mistrust in Niger and the U.S., from everyday doubts about healers and medicines to accelerating skepticism or rejection of biomedicine, public health, pandemic responses, and governments. I will argue that Nigériens' and Americans' perspectives on medical mistrust have much in common despite considerable historical, socioeconomic, and cultural differences, and that we might learn some valuable lessons from each other.

# Taking Mistrust Seriously:
# Living with Uncertainty in Chaotic Times

During my last round of fieldwork, General Abdourahmane Tchiani deposed Mohamed Bazoum, the elected president of Niger, via a bloodless coup d'état on July 26, 2023. One evening a few days after the coup I was enjoying conversation with a friend, Ibrahim, on the veranda of the house that I was renting. Ibrahim, referring to the region, declared while laughing, "Everyone is their own government."[1] He explained that the phrase did not merely refer to the recent political upheaval, but rather to much deeper, longstanding problems regarding the functioning of governments. It means if one wants reliable electricity, one needs to install a generator or solar panels. If one wants reliable water, one needs to drill a borehole and purchase storage containers. If one wants health care, one needs a community of family, friends, and contacts to help with advice and funding for it. That he could laugh about it is a good example of how West Africans use humor to deal with difficult situations. As we were talking the power went out but within seconds the house's generator engaged, and we both remarked that we were very fortunate to have one while much of the middle-class neighborhood remained dark.

Over the previous couple of days and for many months afterward, many of my poorer friends told me that "We are in the dark with mosquitoes." This was the result of one of the first sanctions imposed on Niger because of the coup—Nigeria, which provided Niger with three-quarters of its electricity, cut off supplies.[2] Niger's challenges did not end there. Nigeria and Benin, also as part of ECOWAS sanctions, closed their borders with Niger. This led to shortages and rising prices of medicines and food in Niger since significant amounts of basic consumer goods in Niger arrive in coastal ports and move overland through Benin and Nigeria. The poor disproportionately suffered, as is often the case with economic sanctions. After seven months, ECOWAS sanctions on Niger were finally lifted in late February 2024, two weeks before the beginning of Ramadan, which fell during the hot season in Niger for the second consecutive year.[3]

During this crisis, Nigériens relied on themselves and on sharing information, medicine, and financial resources with each other for health care because, as my friend had said, "everyone is their own government." Some evidence suggests that this was a boon for traditional and Islamic healers using locally sourced medicines, even though most Nigériens had less money to spend during the period of sanctions than before them, because it was primarily pharmaceutical drugs that were being blocked from entry into Niger by the sanctions.[4] Most Nigériens, even those who can afford only one meal a day, will offer to share it when friends appear as they are sitting down to eat. Life is difficult for Nigériens, but it would be so much more difficult without their ethic of cooperation and sharing.

These added challenges are new, but they come on top of other difficulties that have long fostered Nigériens' mistrust of their government and the medical establishment. This long history is partly why medical mistrust must be taken seriously in Niger and everywhere. Lessons about health, healing, and medical mistrust from Niger shed light on what it means to live in a global era of intersecting precarities, suspicion, counterfeits, fake news, post-truth, and artificial intelligence. I argue that we must relinquish thinking of mistrust and trust as dichotomous opposites and instead think of a mistrust–trust continuum and the coexistence of mistrust and trust. For example, Nigérien men mistrust women as the source of heat–cold imbalance and yet men primarily trust women healers to treat it. Mistrust and trust operate in tandem, and it is precisely the ambiguity and uncertainty that open spaces where future therapies can be contemplated. Pervasive skepticism and mistrust persist even after Nigériens have been successfully treated; especially if they used medicines from multiple sectors simultaneously, they may not be confident about which one(s) worked. Furthermore, medicines come and go frequently in Niger. Nigériens often find medicines that they think are efficacious only to be frustrated later when they are no longer available, bringing them back to square one.

Mistrust and trust are complexly contextual, nuanced, and relational, involving affective dimensions (emotion, attitude) and cognitive dimensions (knowledge, perception). People of different classes, genders, ethnicities, "races," ages, occupations, education, and locations experience and respond to uncertainty and mistrust differently because mistrust is embedded in histories and cultures. Mistrust and trust can only be understood holistically. A single Nigérien may exhibit mistrust differently depending on social, political, and economic context. For example, Mamadou, the traditional bonesetter, joined his friends in deriding *bokaye* even though he is a sort of *boka* himself in that he uses esoteric magic in his therapies. Mamadou generally mistrusted biomedicine and never used it but referred his friend Aboubacar to a hospital to treat his paralysis after his own efforts to help Aboubacar failed.

Mistrust serves as a pragmatic, "defensive arrangement" (Luhmann 2014, 1) in contexts of great uncertainty. It leads to engagement with complexity and thinking about and choosing alternatives. Furthermore, mistrust is shared and spreads through language (stories and rumors) creating fluid "communities of mistrust." Mistrust is inadvertently productive in that it leads to multiple therapeutic options for patients while leaving plenty of openings for healers. Because Nigériens mistrust healers and medicines they regularly seek new ones. Furthermore, it is relatively easy to get started as an Islamic pharmacist and very easy to begin working as a street pharmaceutical healer. Both are constantly bringing new products to the streets of Niamey, including medicines that Nigériens did not know they needed, as it were. I also interrogated and complicated a range of other dichotomies, including health–illness, heat–cold, patient–healer, and a trichotomy—traditional–Islamic–biomedical. In short, mistrust significantly shapes Nigériens' lives and choices in medicine and beyond and thus merits serious attention.

*Negotiating Mistrust* established the prevalence of medical mistrust in Niamey, its historical roots, and the ways that patients navigate mistrust as well as strategies used by healers to overcome mistrust. Niger is a unique place; however, many scholars emphasize that in today's world medical mistrust—and mistrust in general—is universal and building momentum on a global scale. Scoones (2019, 5) argues that "Uncertainty defines our times," and that uncertainties are accelerating across all domains of life. Mühlfried (2018, 16, 20) similarly asserts that we are living in a "post-truth" era defined by "loss of trust in experts" and "loss of faith in 'truth' . . . and where mistrust-driven sentiments are valued higher than objective evidence." For example, in the U.S. politicians are making public health decisions that conflict with the advice of public health experts; in many rural areas of the U.S. people are deeply mistrustful of university professors; and conspiracy theories and deliberate misinformation proliferate. Bauman (2007) describes the contemporary moment as "liquid times," an era in which "life is shifting, mobile, provisional, and improvised" (Scoones 2019, 11–12), akin to the "zigzagging" described by Masquelier (2019, 186).

Americans may learn from Nigériens on the periphery of the global economy who live with extensive experience of mistrust, ambiguity, intersecting precarities, structural violence, and for whom "confronting uncertainty is therefore a way of life, not a problem to overcome" (Scoones 2019, 12). Niger and the U.S might appear to have absolutely nothing in common as the former is one of poorest countries in the world whereas the latter is the richest country in the world. However, Nigériens and Americans share a pervasive and accelerating mistrust of medical professionals, science, news, and government. This transpires on an everyday basis and is also starkly revealed during times of crisis like the COVID-19 pandemic. Just as Nigériens are often overwhelmed by the dozens of ever-changing health options in three major medical sectors on the streets of Niamey, Americans are bombarded with direct-to-consumer advertising of pharmaceuticals in one of only two countries in the world that permit it.[5] Direct-to-consumer advertising also creates a different dynamic of mistrust among physicians in the U.S. who now must contend with patients demanding prescriptions for drugs that they have seen advertised on television and threatening to find physicians who will provide them if they do not comply. Furthermore, Americans can now access and utilize a proliferating variety of alternatives to biomedicine, including Chinese medicine, crystals, cannabis, and traditional medicines of Niger such as moringa leaf, among many others. Nigériens and Americans are often deeply mistrustful of many the medical options that exist in their countries even as they demand more and more options. The two attitudes work together. Mistrust of medicine leads people to demand alternatives, while ever-increasing medical possibilities in turn fuel skepticism.

The prevalence of mistrust in Niger and elsewhere means that medical mistrust is a critical component of everyday health care, public health policy, and pandemic preparedness in Niger and the U.S. and thus must be factored into decision-making on all these fronts. While I have emphasized the logic, pragmatism, and productivity of medical mistrust, I also recognize that medical mistrust can be incredibly frustrating for Nigériens as well as American patients who want to trust their health care providers, and that medical mistrust can have lethal consequences for public health, especially during epidemics and pandemics. On a quotidian basis, the efficacy of the medicines sold by the traditional, Islamic, and pharmaceutical healers on the streets of

Niamey is hotly debated by Nigériens who think that good medicines can also be lethal if used improperly. Parallel debates occur in the U.S.

Niamey's informal-sector healers really know how to listen; show empathy, respect, and friendliness; and make themselves figuratively and literally accessible to their patients. Only a minority of physicians receive substantial training in communication skills with patients in the U.S., where it not required, and even fewer receive intercultural communication training. Miscommunication and ineffective communication are major sources of mistrust in the U.S., especially in ethnically discordant healer–patient interactions (Boyas and Valera 2011). Physicians and other health care professionals in the U.S. might overcome some of their patients' mistrust with more serious training and by following the practice of the street healers of Niamey. Street healers communicate effectively with patients in Niger because they take their mistrust seriously, know that they need to work to win patients' trust, and recognize that many medical alternatives are available. If physicians in the U.S. take patients' mistrust seriously, they can alleviate it.

The COVID-19 pandemic led to enormous worldwide suffering and seven million premature deaths. State and global policies designed to mitigate the spread of the virus saved many lives while simultaneously severely disrupting peoples' lives and upending local and global economies. Niger's situation and Nigérien perceptions of COVID-19 are unique. Nevertheless, the Niger case may offer some broad lessons for comparative analysis. For example, in the U.S., where biomedicine enjoys as much hegemony as anyplace in the world and more than 1.2 million people succumbed to the disease. COVID-19 rapidly became highly politicized and right-wing politicians and activists openly express hostility to vaccinations, mask-wearing, and physical distancing. In a typical example, a writer in my local paper matter-of-factly declared that "Vaccines cause autism, ADHD, childhood cancers, diabetes, eczema, and epilepsy" (Rogers 2024, 14). In the U.S. less than 70 percent of people finished the initial two-dose vaccination series in 2021, and less than 20 percent received the bivalent booster shot in 2022. While these are considerably higher vaccination rates than Nigériens,' given the virulence and transmissibility of COVID-19 in the U.S. the tens of millions of Americans who ignored public health policies contributed to hundreds of thousands of preventable deaths. Notably, this is transpiring in a context of steadily eroding confidence in science, corporations (especially "Big Pharma"), and the government in the U.S., just as is happening in Niger.

Similarly, the rumors that Nigériens in Niamey are sharing about COVID-19 as a plot to sterilize Africans and Muslims as "weapons of the weak," and the behaviors that resulted have the potential to lead to catastrophic consequences—for example, if a highly contagious variant of COVID-19 were to arrive in Niger or another pandemic strikes there. Although it was pressured by the WHO and other international agencies to impose a wide range of restrictions, it appears that the Nigérien state made a well-intended effort to protect Nigériens. But since so few Nigériens trust international institutions or their government and there was no evident crisis, the messaging was largely rejected. In terms of pandemic preparedness and response, public health workers in Niger must find pragmatic and respectful ways of engaging with people who are most trusted by Nigériens, especially religious leaders. This is critical though easier said than done, but not impossible with respectful, culturally sensitive, and pragmatic approaches (Farmer 2003; Harrison and Wu 2020). Parallel approaches in the U.S, tailored to specific communities known to mistrust and reject state public health measures merit consideration.

Public health workers are more likely to gain the trust of Nigériens and Americans if they pay more attention to local cultural values and norms and apply lessons learned in past situations. For example, based on their belief that the polio vaccine was contaminated with sterilization agents, "In 2003, political and religious leaders in four largely Muslim states in northern Nigeria called on parents not to cooperate with the polio immunization drive launched by the Global Polio Eradication Initiative (GPEI) of the World Health Organization and carried out by the Nigerian Ministry of Health in co-operation with UNICEF" (Kaler 2009, 1,712). Similar rejection of polio immunizations occurred just across the border in southern Niger (Masquelier 2012; Sams and Hrynick 2020). The vaccination campaign was resumed after a 16-month stoppage only when the Supreme Council for Sharia in Nigeria "and the Nigerian state were finally able to reach a compromise by agreeing to procure vaccines only from companies in Islamic countries, and to test those vaccines for the presence of contraceptives and other toxins" (Kaler 2009, 1,712). It is plausible that Nigériens would be more likely to accept COVID-19 tests and vaccinations—and other vaccines in the future—if they were manufactured and tested in Muslim countries and distributed by the Red Crescent. Parallel approaches might be effective with subcultures in the U.S. Serious, respectful engagement with people's mistrust that emphasizes persuasion over coercion can help overcome medical mistrust (R. Idrissa 2021; Sams and

Hrynick 2020). Rather than being dismissive of and condescending toward people's health decisions—such as rejecting vaccinations—it is important to investigate and make sense of why people make certain choices in particular contexts. Understanding their medical mistrust, mistrust of government, and the links between them could help shape policies that lead to safer behaviors.

Medical mistrust shapes Nigériens' decisions and lives. However, they are not paralyzed by medical mistrust. Instead Nigériens relentlessly pursue health and well-being and strive to survive with dignity in a context of intense uncertainty and intersecting precarities. Niger cut its 2024 budget by 40 percent due to international sanctions and the withdrawal of Western aid in the wake of the 2023 coup d'état. This book's focus on the ways Nigériens navigate medical pluralism and medical mistrust in the informal sector is particularly relevant at this juncture and for the near future, because state budget cuts will inevitably further weaken Niger's already inadequate formal-sector health care infrastructure and thus amplify the importance of informal- sector healing.

# NOTES

## Introduction

1. This example illustrates the fluidity of ethnicity in Niger. I use the ethnic terms that are used by the people I interviewed. I discuss this theme in more detail in Chapter 1.

2. One USD was equivalent to 500 West African Communauté Financière Africaine (CFA) francs during my research from 2017 to 2023. It is used by eight West African countries.

3. These include Abdalla 1992, Etkin 1992, Heller 2019, C. Idrissa 2023, Jaffré and Olivier de Sardan 2023, Masquelier 2019b, Moussa 2023, Olivier de Sardan 1998, Renne 2010, Stock 1981, Stoller 1989, Stoller and Olkes 1987, Wall 1988, and Youngstedt 2021.

4. See Casey 2021, Heller 2019, Masquelier 2001, Moussa 2023.

5. See Loftsdóttir 2008.

6. See Casey 2021, Etkin 1992, Last 1992, Sams 2017, Stock 1981, Wall 1988.

7. See Masquelier 2001.

8. See Olivier de Sardan 1998, Stoller 1989, Stoller and Olkes 1987.

9. See Rasmussen 2001.

10. See Popenoe 2004.

11. See Last 1992, Loftsdóttir 2008, Masquelier 2001, Popenoe 2004, Rasmussen 2001, Stoller 1989, Stoller and Olkes 1987.

12. See Cooper 2019, Heller 2019, Moussa 2023.

13. See Heller 2019.

14. See Renne 2010.

15. See Casey 2021, Masquelier 2001, Rasmussen 1995, Stoller 1989, Stoller and Olkes 1987.

16. Zarma and Songhay are slightly different ethnic groups, though they speak dialects of the same language and are sometimes rereferred to as Zarma-Songhay or Songhay-Zarma, as I do in this book. In Niamey, Zarma outnumber Songhay by roughly nine to one.

17. Niger's ethnic composition includes 53 percent Hausa, 21 percent Zarma-Songhay, 11 percent Tuareg, 6.5 percent Fulani, 6.5 percent Kanuri, and several other small groups (Index Mundi 2022).

## Chapter 1

1. The structural adjustment programs imposed by the World Bank and the International Monetary Fund across Africa and the Global South required countries to reduce spending on public health care and introduced user fees. These policies led to widespread suffering, especially among the poorest people. This problem has been extensively documented (Prince and Marsland 2014).

2. Abdalla 1992; Baronov 2008; Bierlich 1999; Cooper 2019; Hunt 1999; Idrissa 2023; Janzen 1978; Olsen and Sargent 2017; Rasmussen 2001; Roberts 2021; Twumasi 1979.

3. Crandon-Malamud 1991; Heemskerk et al. 2022.

4. Uvulectomies, involving the surgical excision of the uvula by traditional healers, are practiced in many African countries, including those in the Maghreb (Prual et al. 1994, 1077) as well as Cameroon, Ethiopia, Niger, Nigeria, and Tanzania (Lange and Mfaume 2022, 2). In a survey of children in Niamey, Prual et al. (1994, 1077) found that 20 percent had undergone uvulectomies. It is particularly prevalent among some Hausa communities of Niger who perform the surgery a few days just before or during naming ceremonies on the seventh day after the birth of babies. They think that this prevents the potential swelling of the uvula that could lead to suffocation (Prual et al. 1994, 1078; Wall 1988, 185). Many of my interlocutors offered this explanation as well. Hausa, Zarma, and other ethnic groups also use uvulectomies as "a curative practice, both for children and adults, for vomiting, diarrhea, anorexia, the child's rejection of the breast, growth retardation, and fever" (Prual et al. 1994, 1078). Some uvulectomy patients in Niger (Prual et al. 1994, 1078), Nigeria (Wall 1988, 185), and Tanzania (Lange and Mfaume 2022, 13) are taken to hospitals with severe complications such as infections and hemorrhaging that can be fatal.

5. Bloodletting is used in Niger to remove "dead blood" that causes lethargy and other problems. The procedure involves making small incisions, usually on the back, and then creating a vacuum by cupping the area with a small cow's horn that has a small hole on the tip.

6. It is estimated that 96 percent of Nigérien males have been circumcised (Morris et al. 2016). Typically, it occurs when boys are about six years old. My interviewees explained matter-of-factly that male circumcision is required in Islam. Traditional barber-surgeons perform the surgery. Although they usually identify as Muslim, they are not credentialed by Muslim institutions. Hence, circumcision illustrates the intertwining of traditional and Islamic health practices.

7. Less than 2 percent of females have undergone female cutting or female genital mutilation in Niger, where it has been illegal since 2003 (UNICEF 2019, 2).

8. The duality in the power of healers—a good side and a "dark side"—is a theme that is evident elsewhere in West Africa (Gottlieb 1989, 254).

9. This problem has been extensively documented across West Africa. See, for example, Gottlieb (2004) and Jaffré and Olivier de Sardan (2003).

## Chapter 2

1. Feminist legal scholars (MacKinnon 1979) have long recognized the emotional cost of labor for women facing sexual harassment while working—even the subtle forms of harassment endured by women selling heat medicine on the streets of Niamey.

2. The most serious problem with the informal market in pharmaceuticals may involve antibiotic misuse, including overprescription (or mis-prescription) for a wide range of nonbacterial infections, as well as under-prescription in the form of selling or consuming less than full courses of antibiotics. The *akwaku* (informal-sector pharmaceutical healers) and their clients are potentially contributing to a local and global health crisis of antibiotic resistant bacteria. In their global survey of the overuse of antibiotics, Blaser et al. (2021, 2) document that, "between 2000 and 2015, antibiotic consumption increased . . . 77% . . . among LMICs [low and middle-income countries]" where well over one-half of antibiotics are sold without prescriptions by untrained vendors. Niger, like most countries, has laws against this, but they are rarely enforced.

## Chapter 3

1. Heller (2019, 134, 135) explains that "the real price of free care" was that these reforms "without any supporting accompanying measures . . . nearly resulted in the collapse of the whole health system."

2. "The Human Development Index (HDI) is a summary measure of average achievement in key dimensions of human development: a long and healthy life [measured by life expectancy at birth], being knowledgeable [measured by mean years of education of those over 25 years] and having a decent standard of living [measured by Gross National Income per capita]. The HDI is the geometric mean of normalized indices for each of the three dimensions" (UNDP 2022).

3. See Idrissa (2017) and Thurston (2018) for more detailed discussion of insecurity in the region.

4. My analysis of the medical mistrust–trust nexus draws from, applies, and aims to extend three bodies of literature. This includes first, anthropological (Carey 2017; Mühlfried 2018; Mühlfried 2019) and sociological (Luhmann 1993; Sztompka 1999) theories of mistrust and trust. Florian Mühlfried's edited volume, *Mistrust: Ethnographic Approximations* (2018), and his book, *Mistrust: A Global Perspective* (2019), in particular have sharpened my thinking about mistrust and its relation to trust. Although Mühlfried focuses on general social theory and its applications to political situations, his ideas can fruitfully by applied to enhance understanding medical mistrust and trust. Second, I refer to a global range of studies by medical anthropologists of medical mistrust and trust, including in the U.S. (Boyas and Valera 2011; Jaiswal and Haliitis 2019), in Italy (Pasquini 2023), and in Turkey (Sengul and Bulut 2020). Third, I draw from the literature on health and healing in Niger, almost all of which considers medical mistrust, especially mistrust of biomedicine (e.g., Cooper 2019; Heller 2019; R. Idrissa 2021; Jaffré and Olivier de Sardan 2003; Masquelier 2012; Rasmussen 2001; Sams and Hrynick 2020).

5. I have used this broad generalization to make a point. In practice today, much of the medicine consumed in rural Niger is purchased with cash at local markets, and family and friends commonly share medicines in Niamey.

6. Forty-six percent of Nigérien men over the age of 15 are literate in French, while only 30 percent of Nigérien women over the age of 15 are literate in French (World Bank Group 2023). Alidou (2024, 25) indicates that in Niger literacy rates in Arabic are lower than in French, and that the gendered literacy gap in Arabic is greater that the gendered literacy gap in French.

## Chapter 4

1. These included Captopril + HCT Denk and Lasilix Faible, which are standard pharmaceuticals for treating high blood pressure.

## Chapter 5

1. See van der Geest and Whyte (1999); van der Geest, Whyte, and Hardon (1996); and Whyte, van der Geest, and Hardon (2002).

2. There may be some exceptions to this generalization. My understanding is that illicit drugs in Niamey circulate in hidden, very discreet circles of people.

3. Five of the 11 who did not inherit this job apprenticed with healers outside of their ethnic groups, including four Zarma men who studied with Hausa healers and a Tuareg who learned from Fulani friends. This cross-cultural medical training is another example of *brassage*.

4. These prices vary considerably, because healers of each sector offer a variety of different medicines for treating malaria.

5. I simultaneously do not want to overstate the importance of this association. All the traditional healers in the sample are aware of ATPN and know that it is recognized by the state; however, only 12 of the 42 in my sample are members.

6. Among Nigériens, "the bush" refers to wild, uncultivated land. Many Nigériens living in rural areas collect their own medicinal plants and rely on traditional healers for only their most complicated illnesses.

7. Honey is used to treat cuts and scrapes, typhoid, and stomach and liver ailments. Dates are particularly beneficial for pregnant women and their fetuses and provides protection again poison and sorcery. Olive oil is thought to prevent various forms of cancer and to alleviate high blood pressure. Islamic healers use ginger to treat respiratory problems, arthritis, impotence, and to prevent blood clots and strengthen the heart. Black cumin seeds, or *habbatus sauda*, strengthen the immune system. Islamic healers of Niamey regularly quote the Prophet Muhammad, who said, "*habbatus sauda* can cure every disease except death."

8. There are multiple, gendered types of "Muslim attire" in Niger, and fashion trends change over time. See Masquelier (2013) and Rasmussen (2013) for detailed discussion.

9. See R. Idrissa (2017) for an excellent discussion of the history of the Izala movement.

10. Susan M. O'Brien (2001, 224) explained that *ruk'ya* is an ancient form of Islamic exorcism that was introduced in Kano in the late 1990s. It sometimes involves a violent approach including Qur'anic recitation to expel spirits. However, *ruk'ya* generated some controversy because "The newly adopted Islamic methods mirror *bori* therapeutics and depart from the most common Islamic approaches to spirit afflictions in northern Nigeria, in that they induce possession and negotiate with spirits as part of the healing process" (O'Brien 2001, 224).

11. Increasing numbers of Nigériens are learning English, but less than 2 percent are literate in English. The same is true of literacy in Hausa (and other Nigérien languages), which—with few exceptions—have never been taught in Nigérien schools.

12. I attempted to contact a few Islamic chemists of Kano to understand the rationales behind these labels, but I was unsuccessful.

13. Other Hausa terms for itinerant drug vendors include *masu talla magunguna* (those displaying medicines for sale) or *masu sai da magunguna* (medicine sellers). The Zarma term is *safarikoy* (medicine vendor). Some Nigériens use the French terms *médecin par terre* (street doctor) and *médicament de la rue* (street medicine) or simply *pharmacie* to gain the attention of a mobile drug vendor.

14. Twenty percent indicated that they entered the trade upon receiving advice from other *akwaku*—typically older brothers and uncles—or by imitating other *akwaku*. Four of the 60 *akwaku* reported that they chose this work because it is easy and does not require literacy.

## Chapter 6

1. Many Nigériens suspect that COVID-19 deaths were overcounted, especially during the initial months of the crisis. A young Hausa man explained, "Hospitals automatically suspected that everyone who died then had died of the coronavirus." In contrast, it is likely that cases of COVID-19 and deaths due to COVID-19 are being undercounted, as several of the people with whom I spoke and interviewed believed. The explanation that "A majority of Nigériens do not want to get tested when they have COVID-19 symptoms, and even when they do there is a lack of health centers for testing," was typical. Furthermore, very few autopsies are performed in Niger, and most Nigériens are buried within 24–48 hours of death per Muslim practice.

2. I referred to examples of when people advised me against taking Nigérien traditional medicines on the grounds that they are not suitable for White people and could harm me.

3. I also suggest that it may not be a stretch to argue that negative reaction to Nigérien state COVID-19 policies played an important role in the government's demise and/or in the popular support for General Tchiani after his coup d'état on July 26, 2023 toppled Niger's democratically elected government. President Mahamadou Issoufou was in office when the pandemic begun and avidly pushed the public health mandates that so angered people, but it was Mohamed Bazoum, his essentially handpicked successor who came to power in April 2021, who was actually deposed.

4. No official explanation for this discrepancy was offered, as far as I know. One explanation could be that since Christians make up at most 1 percent of Nigériens their numbers were too small to matter. This, of course, makes no sense in terms of public health because Nigérien churches are densely crowded during services that could have become super-spreader events. It is not difficult to imagine ways that this policy may have inspired rumors or may have been influenced by them. Perhaps the state did not care about Christians, or perhaps the state was demonstrating more concern for Christians' rights than Muslims' rights. I have very few connections in Christian communities in Niger, and hence I am unaware of their perspectives on COVID-19 and state policies.

## Conclusion

1. I did not know it at the time, but learned later that this term is commonly used throughout Nigeria. See Smith (2022).

2. Only about 5 percent of Nigériens in Niamey can afford generators and the diesel fuel to run them regularly. A majority can afford only enough electricity to power a few light bulbs and fans.

3. On March 11, 2024, the first full day of Ramadan, temperatures in Niamey reached 111 degrees Fahrenheit. Comparable high temperatures persisted throughout Ramadan and into May.

4. This evidence comes from personal communication with trusted contacts in Niamey, and I argue that it makes sense.

5. New Zealand is the other country where direct-to-consumer advertising of prescription pharmaceuticals is permitted.

# REFERENCES

Abdalla, Ismail H. 1992. "Diffusion of Islamic Medicine into Hausaland." In *The Social Basis of Health and Healing in Africa*, edited by Steven Feierman and John M. Janzen, 177–94. Berkeley: University of California Press.

AFP. 2020. "Sahel: Niger faces escalating riots in coming days." *The North Africa Journal*. April 22, 2020. Accessed June 4, 2020. https://north-africa.com/2020/04/sahel-niger-faces-escalating-riots-in-coming-days/.

Alhassan, Aliyu. 2022. "Modern Islamic Medicine and Modern Islamic Health Centers in Kano Metropolis,1988 to 2012." *Journal for the International Society for the History of Islamic Medicine* 21 (42): 10–17.

Alidou, Ousseina D. 2005. *Engaging Modernity: Muslim Women and the Politics of Agency in Postcolonial Niger*. Madison: University of Wisconsin Press.

———. 2024. *Protest Arts, Gender, and Social Change: Fiction, Popular Songs, and the Media in Hausa Society Across Borders*. Ann Arbor: University of Michigan Press.

Appadurai, Arjun. 1986. *The Social Life of Things: Commodities in Cultural Perspective*. Cambridge: Cambridge University Press.

Archibong, Belinda, and Francis Annan. 2021. "What do Pfizer's 1996 drug trials in Nigeria teach us about vaccine hesitancy?" *Africa in Focus*, December 3, 2021. Accessed December 23, 2021. https://www.brookings.edu/blog/africa-in-focus/2021/12/03/what-do-pfizers-1996-drug-trials-in-nigeria-teach-us-about-vaccine-hesitancy/.

Atuire, Caesar A., Grace Addison, Samuel Asiedu Owusu, and Patricia Kingori. 2021. "'Covid Cure (1)': Anas's Investigative Journalism and the Ethics of Uncovering Fakes in African Spaces." *Journal of African Cultural Studies* 33 (3): 312–19.

Baronov, David. 2008. *The African Transformation of Western Medicine and the Dynamics of Global Cultural Exchange*. Philadelphia: Temple University Press.

Barrère, M., I. A. Kourguéni, and S. Attama. 1999. "Fécondité, planification familiale et santé de la mère et de l'enfant au Niger: Situation régionale." Niamey: CARE International and Calverton, MD: Macro International.

Bauman, Zygmunt. 2007. *Liquid Times: Living in an Age of Uncertainty*. Cambridge: Polity Press.

Baxerres, Carine. 2001. "Pourquoi un marché informel médicaments dans les pays francophones d'Afrique?" *Éditions Karthala* 123: 117–36.

Ben Ahmed, Lassad. 2020. "Niger / COVID-19: Des manifestations contre certaines mesures de restriction." *Agence Anadolu*, April 20, 2020. Accessed January 12, 2022. https://www.aa.com.tr/fr/afrique/niger-covid-19-des-manifestations-contre-certaines-mesures-de-restriction/1811804.

Bernus, Suzanne. 1969. *Particularismes Ethnique en Milieu Urbain: L'Example de Niamey.* Paris: Université de Paris, Institut d'Ethnologie, Musée de l'Homme.

Blaser, Martin J., Melissa K. Melby, Margaret Lock, and Mark Nichter. 2021. "Accounting for Variation in and Overuse of Antibiotics Among Humans." *BioEssays* 43 (2): e2000163. https://doi.org/10.1002/bies.202000163.

Boyas, Javier, and Pamela A. Valera. 2011. "Determinants of Trust in Medical Personnel." *Hispanic Health Care International* 9 (3): 144–52.

Campbell, Donald. 2013. *Arabian Medicine and its Influence on the Middle Ages,* Vol. 1. Originally published 1926. London: Routledge.

Carey, Matthew. 2017. *Mistrust: An Ethnographic Theory.* Chicago: University of Chicago Press.

Casey, Conerly. 2021. "Eco-intimacy and spirit exorcism in the Nigerian Sahel." *The Senses and Society* 16 (2): 132–50.

Cooper, Barbara M. 2006. *Evangelical Christians in the Muslim Sahel.* Bloomington: Indiana University Press.

———. 2019. *Countless Blessings: A History of Childbirth and Reproduction in the Sahel.* Bloomington: Indiana University Press.

Crandon-Malamud, Libbet. 1991. *From the Fat of Our Souls: Social Change, Political Process, and Medical Pluralism in Bolivia.* Berkeley: University of California Press.

Dogru, Alaattin. 2020. "Niger's labor minister dies from COVID-19." *Agence Anadolu,* May 5, 2020. Accessed January 14, 2022, https://www.aa.com.tr/en/africa/niger-s-labor-minister-dies-from-covid-19-tv/1829129.

Douglas, Mary. 1992. *Risk and Blame: Essays in cultural theory.* London: Routledge.

Etkin, Nina L. 1992. "'Side Effects': Cultural Constructions and Reinterpretations of Western Pharmaceuticals." *Medical Anthropology Quarterly* 6 (2): 99–113.

Etkin, Nina L., Paul J. Ross, and Ibrahim Muazzamu. 1990. "The Indigenization of Pharmaceuticals: Therapeutic Transitions in Rural Hausaland." *Social Science and Medicine* 30 (8): 919–28.

Evans-Pritchard, E. E. 1937. *Witchcraft, Oracles, and Magic Among the Azande.* Oxford: Clarendon Press.

Falen, Douglas J. 2018. *African Science: Witchcraft, Vodun, and Healing in Southern Benin.* Madison: University of Wisconsin Press.

Farmer, Paul. 2003. *Pathologies of Power: Health, Human Rights, and the New War on the Poor.* Berkeley: University of California Press.

———. 2010. "Landmine Boy and Stupid Deaths." In *Partner to the Poor: A Paul Farmer Reader,* edited by Haun Saussy, 409–22. Berkeley: University of California Press.

Fatunde, O. J., and J. B. Familusi. 2001. "Injection-induced sciatic nerve injury in Nigerian children." *Central African Journal of Medicine* 47 (2): 35–38.

Faucon, Benoit. 2021. "Niger Is the Land That Covid-19 Forgot." *Wall Street Journal,* July 17, 2021. Accessed July 29, 2021. https://www.wsj.com/articles/niger-is-the-land-thatcovid-19forgot-11626531245.

Feierman, Steven, and John M. Janzen. 1992. "Introduction." In *The Social Basis of Health and Healing in Africa,* edited by Steven Feierman and John M. Janzen, 1–24. Berkeley: University of California Press.

Frazer, James G. 1922. *The Golden Bough: A Study in Magic and Religion.* New York: Macmillan.

Fuglestad, Finn. 1983. *A History of Niger 1850–1960.* Cambridge: Cambridge University Press.

Gado, Boureïma Alpha. 1997. *Niamey: Garin kaptan Salma (Histoire d'une ville)*. Niamey: Nouvelle Imprimerie du Niger.

Geschiere, Peter. 1997. *The Modernity of Witchcraft*. Charlottesville: University of Virginia Press.

Geschiere, Peter, and Cyprian Fisiy. 1994. "Domesticating Personal Violence: Witchcraft, Courts and Confessions in Cameroon." *Africa* 64 (3): 323–41.

Gottlieb, Alma. 1989. "Witches, Kings, and the Sacrifice of Identity; or, The Power of Paradox and the Paradox of Power among the Beng of Ivory Coast." In *Creativity of Power: Cosmology and Action in African Societies*, edited by W. Arens and Ivan Karp, 245–72. Washington, DC: Smithsonian Institution Press.

———. 2004. *The Afterlife Is Where We Come from: The Culture of Infancy in West Africa*. Chicago: University of Chicago Press.

———. 2008. "Loggers vs. Spirits in the Beng Forest, Côte d'Ivoire: Competing Models." In *African Sacred Groves: Ecological Dynamics and Social Change*, edited by Michael J. Sheridan and Celia Nyamweru, 149–63. Athens: Ohio University Press.

Greenwood, Bernard. 1992. "Cold or Spirits? Ambiguity and Syncretism in Moroccan Therapeutics." In *The Social Basis of Health and Healing in Africa*, edited by Steven Feierman and John M. Janzen, 285–314. Berkeley: University of California Press.

Halliburton, Murphy. 2017. *India and the Patent Wars*. Ithaca, NY: Cornell University Press.

Hansen, Karen Tranberg, with Anne Line Dalsgaard, Katherine V. Gough, Ulla Ambrosius Madsen, Karen Valentin, and Norbert Wildermuth. 2008. *Youth and the City in the Global South*. Bloomington: Indiana University Press.

Harrison, Emily A., and Julia W. Wu. 2020. "Vaccine confidence in the time of COVID-19. *European Journal of Epidemiology* 35: 325–30.

Heemskerk, Marieke, Francois-Michel Le Tourneau, Helene Hiwat, Hedley Cairo, and Pierre Pratley. 2022. "In a life full of risks, COVID-19 makes little difference: Responses to COVID-19 among mobile migrants in Suriname and French Guiana." *Social Science & Medicine* 296: 114747.

Heller, Alison. 2019. *Fistula Politics: Birthing Injuries and the Quest for Continence in Niger*. New Brunswick, NJ: Rutgers University Press.

iciniger.com. 2018. Niger: importante saisie de 29 tonnes de produits pharmaceutiques prohibés. Accessed October 12, 2018. http://iciniger.com/niger-importante-saisie-de-29-tonnes-de-produits-pharmaceutiques-prohibés/.

Idrissa, Cheifou. 2021. "La survenue de la crise de la COVID-19 au Niger." Unpublished report. Niamey.

———. 2023. "La pharmacopée traditionnelle et les pharmacies islamiques au Niamey." Unpublished report. Niamey.

Idrissa, Rahmane. 2017. *The Politics of Islam in the Sahel: Between Persuasion and Violence*. New York: Routledge.

———. 2020. *Historical Dictionary of Niger*. 5th ed. Lanham, MD: Rowman & Littlefield.

———. 2021. "Niger in the year of the COVID-19 pandemic: The fear, the grief, the coping." Include Knowledge Platform on Inclusive Development Policies. Think Tank Économie Politique et Gouvernance Autonome. Niamey.

Idowu. O. A., A. E. Ogunrinu, A. Akinremi, O. E. Aladeyelu, B. Kaka, and J. K. Adelugba. 2011. "Injection Induced Sciatic Nerve Injury among Children Managed in a Nigerian Physiotherapy Clinic: A Five Year Review." *African Journals Online (AJPARS)* 3 (1): 13–16.

Igun, U. A. 1987. "Why We Seek Treatment Here: Retail Pharmacy and Clinical Treatment in Maiduguri, Nigeria." *Social Science & Medicine* 24 (8): 689–95.

Index Mundi. 2022. "Niger Demographics Profile." Accessed August 6, 2024. https://www .indexmundi.com/niger/demographics_profile.html.

Institute for Health Metrics and Evaluation (IHME). 2019. "Niger, 2019." Accessed February 25, 2023. https://www.healthdata.org/niger.

IRACM (Institute of Research Against Counterfeit Medicines). 2019. "Niger: Clandestine Fake Medicines Factory in Niamey," March 12, 2019. Accessed June 11, 2019. https://www.iracm .com/en/2019/03/niger-clandestine-fake-medicines-factory-niamey/

Jaffré, Yannick, and Jean Pierre Olivier de Sardan, eds. 2003. *Une medicine inhospitalière: Les difficiles relations entre soignant et soignés dans cinq capitals d'Afrique de l'Ouest.* Paris: Karthala.

Jaiswal, Jessica, and Perry N. Halkitis. 2019. "Towards a More Inclusive and Dynamic Understanding of Medical Mistrust Informed by Science." *Behavioral Medicine* 45 (2): 79–85.

Janzen, John M. 1978. *The Quest for Therapy in Lower Zaire.* Berkeley: University of California Press.

———. 2017. "Science in the Moral Space of Health and Healing Paradigms in Western Equatorial Africa." In Olsen and Sargent 2017, 90–109.

Kaler, Amy. 2009. "Health interventions and the persistence of rumour: The circulation of sterility stories in African public health campaigns." *Social Science & Medicine* 68: 1711–99.

Keough, Sara Beth, and Scott M. Youngstedt. 2019. *Water, Life, and Profit: Fluid Economies and Cultures of Niamey, Niger.* New York: Berghahn Books.

Kingori, Patricia. 2021. "Unmuting Conversations on Fakes in African Spaces." *Journal of African Cultural Studies* 33 (3): 239–50.

Kleinman, Arthur. 2017. "Afterward." In Olsen and Sargent 2017, 261–64.

Lange, Siri, and Dorcas Mfaume. 2022. "The folk illness *kimeo* and 'traditional' uvulectomy: An ethnomedical study of care seeking for children with cough and weakness in Dar es Salaam." *Journal of Ethnobiology and Ethnomedicine* 18, 35. https://doi.org/10.1186/s13002 -022-00533-9.

Last, Murray. 1992. "The Importance of Knowing About Not Knowing." In *The Social Basis of Health and Healing in Africa*, edited by Steven Feierman and John M. Janzen, 393–406. Berkeley: University of California Press.

———. 2011. "Another geography: risks to health as perceived in a deep-rural environment in Hausaland." *Anthropology and Medicine* 18 (2): 217–29.

———. 2019. "Medical Ethnography over Time: Penetrating 'the fog of health' in a Nigerian community, 1970–2017." *Anthropology in Action* 26 (1): 52–60.

Last, Murray, and G. L. Chavunduka, eds. 1986. *The Professionalization of African Medicine.* Manchester, U.K.: Manchester University Press.

Lemkin, Rob, dir. 2020. *African Apocalypse.* Devon, UK: Inside Out Films and LemKino Pictures, 2020.

Loftsdóttir, Kristín. 2008. *The Bush Is Sweet: Identity, Power and Development Among WoDaaBe Fulani in Niger.* Uppsala: Nordiska Afrikainstitutet.

Lowes, Robert. 2018. "On the Corner of Happy and Hypocritical: Why is the nation's largest drugstore chain still selling cigarettes?" *The Progressive*, August 1, 2018. Accessed September 10, 2018. progressive.com.

Luhmann, Niklas. 1993. *Risk: A Sociological Theory*. Translated by Rhodes Barrett. New York: Walter de Gruyter.

———. 2014 [1968]. *Vertrauen*. Konstanz, Ger.: UVK.

MacGregor, Hayley, Melissa Leach, Grace Akello, Lawrence Sao Babawo, Moses Baluku, Alice Desclaux, Catherine Grant, Foday Kamara, Fred Martineau, Esther Yei Mokuwa, Melissa Parker, Paul Richards, Kelly Sams, Khodia Sow, and Annie Wilkinson. 2021. "Negotiating Intersecting Precarities: COVID-19, Pandemic Preparedness and Response in Africa." *Medical Anthropology* 41(1): 19–33. https://doi.org/10.1080/01459740.2021.2015591.

MacKinnon, Catharine. 1979. *Sexual Harassment of Working Women: A Case of Sex Discrimination*. New Haven, CT: Yale University Press.

La Maison de l'Artemisia. 2021. "Focus on the Houses of Artemisia in Niger." Accessed October 10, 2023. https://maison-artemisia.org/en/focus-on-the-houses-of-artemisia-in-niger/.

Masquelier, Adeline. 2001. *Prayer Has Spoiled Everything: Possession, Power, and Identity in an Islamic Town of Niger*. Durham, NC: Duke University Press.

———. 2012. "Public Health or Public Threat? Polio Eradication Campaigns, Islamic Revival, and the Materialization of State Power in Niger." In *Medicine, Mobility, and Power in Global Africa*, edited by Hansjörg Dilger, Abdoulaye Kane, and Stacy A. Langwick, 213–40. Bloomington: Indiana University Press.

———. 2013. "Modest Bodies, Stylish Selves: Fashioning Virtue in Niger." In *Veiling in Africa*, edited by Elisha P. Renne, 110–36. Bloomington: Indiana University Press.

———. 2019a. *Fada: Boredom and Belonging in Niger*. Chicago: The University of Chicago Press.

———. 2019b. "Are Spirits Satanic? The Ambiguity of Evil in Niger." In *Engaging Evil: A Moral Anthropology*, edited by William C. Olsen and Thomas J. Csordas, 177–96. New York: Berghahn Books.

———. 2020. "A Matter of Time: Spirit Possession and the Temporalities of School in Niger." *Journal of Africana Religions* 8 (1): 122–45.

Mauss, Marcel. 1954. *The Gift: Form and Reason of Exchange in Archaic Societies*. Translated by W. D. Halls. Original work published 1924. New York: Free Press.

May, John F. 2017. "The Politics of Family Planning Policies and Programs in Sub-Saharan Africa." *Population and Development Review* 43 (S1): 308–29.

Morris, Brian J., Richard G. Wamai, Esther B. Heneberg, Aaron A.R. Tobian, Jeffrey D. Klausner, Joya Banergee, and Catherine A. Haskins. 2016. "Estimation of country-specific and global prevalence of male circumcision: Table 1, Percentage of circumcised males in each of the 237 countries and territories in the world." *Population Health Metrics* 14 (4): 4. doi:10.1186/s12963-016-0073-5.

Moussa, Hadiza. 2023. *Yearning and Refusal: An Ethnography of Female Fertility Management in Niamey, Niger*. Edited by Alice J. Kang and Barbara M. Cooper. Translated by Natalie Kammerer. New York: Oxford University Press.

Mühlfried, Florian. 2018. "Introduction: Approximating Mistrust." In *Mistrust: Ethnographic Approximations*, edited by Florian Mühlfried, 7–22. Beilefeld, Ger.: Verlag.

———. 2019. *Mistrust: A Global Perspective*. Cham, Switz.: Palgrave Macmillan.

Mulemi, Benson A. 2017. "Therapeutic Eclecticism and Cancer Care in a Kenyan Hospital Ward." In Olsen and Sargent 2017, 207–26.

Newman, Paul. 2007. *A Hausa-English Dictionary*. New Haven, CT: Yale University Press.

Niamey.com. 2017. "Niger: saisie de 13 tonnes de médicaments contrefaits en provenance d'Inde." Accessed November 24, 2018. http://news.aniamey.com/h/82647.html

Nowak, Brian. 2018. Personal communication.

———. 2019. Personal communication.

———. 2020. Personal communication.

———. 2021. Personal communication.

O'Brien, Susan M. 2001. "Spirit Discipline: Gender, Islam, and Hierarchies of Treatment in Postcolonial Northern Nigeria." *Interventions: International Journal of Postcolonial Studies* 3 (2): 222–41.

Observer. 2018. "In Niger, unregulated medicine is 'sold like sweets.'" Accessed March 5, 2020. https://observers.france24.com/en/20181221-niger-unregulated-medicine-markets-drugs.

Ogala, George. 2021. "Covid-19, Knowledge Production and the (Un)Making of Truths and Fakes." *Journal of African Cultural Studies* 33 (3): 305–11.

Olivier de Sardan, Jean-Pierre. 1998. "Illness Entities in West Africa." *Anthropology & Medicine* 5 (2): 193–217.

———. 2009. "State Bureaucracy and Governance in West Francophone Africa: An Empirical Diagnosis and Historical Perspective." In *The Governance of Daily Life in Africa: Ethnographic Explorations of Public and Collective Services*, edited by Giorgio Blundo and Pierre-Yves Le Meur, 39–71. Leiden, Neth.: Brill.

Olsen, William C., and Carolyn Sargent, eds. 2017. *African Medical Pluralism*. Bloomington: Indiana University Press.

Ouestafnews. 2021. "Niger : un 'prêt' de 100 mille doses de vaccins AstraZeneca accordé à la Côte d'Ivoire." June 2, 2021. Accessed January 4, 2004. https://www.ouestaf.com/niger-un-pret-de-100-mille-doses-de-vaccins-astrazeneca-accorde-a-la-cote-divoire/.

Our World in Data. 2023. "Niger: Coronavirus Pandemic Country Profile." Accessed December 25, 2023. https://ourworldindata.org/coronavirus/country/niger.

Pasquini, Mirko. 2023. "Mistrustful Dependency: Mistrust as Risk Management in an Italian Emergency Department." *Medical Anthropology* 42 (6): 579–92.

Performance Monitoring for Action (PMA) Niger. 2021. "COVID-19: Résultats de l'enquête de base de la Phase 1, Décembre 2020–Avril 2021."

Popenoe, Rebecca. 2004. *Feeding Desire: Fatness, Beauty, and Sexuality Among a Saharan People.* London: Routledge.

Pouillot, R., C. Bilong, P. Boisier, M. Ciss, A. Moumouni, I. Imani, and P. Nabeth. 2008. "Le circuit informel des médicaments à Yaoundé et à Niamey: Étude de la population des vendeurs et de qualité des médicaments distribués." *Bulletin de la Société de Pathologie Exotique* 101 (2): 113–18.

Prince, Ruth J., and Rebecca Marsland, eds. 2014. *Making and Unmaking Public Health in Africa: Ethnographic and Historical Perspectives.* Athens: Ohio University Press.

Prual, Alain, Youssouf Gamatie, Mariama Djakounda, and Dominique Huguet. 1994. "Traditional uvulectomy in Niger: A public health problem?" *Social Science & Medicine* 39 (8): 1077–82.

Rasmussen, Susan J. 1995. *Spirit Possession and Personhood among the Kel Ewey Tuareg.* Cambridge: Cambridge University Press.

———. 2001. *Healing in Community: Medicine, Contested Terrains, and Cultural Encounters Among the Tuareg.* Westport, CT: Bergin and Garvey.

———. 2013. "Veiling Without Veils: Modesty and Reserve in Tuareg Cultural Encounters." In *Veiling in Africa*, edited by Elisha P. Renne, 34–57. Bloomington: Indiana University Press.

———. 2017. "Spirits and Pills Who Are Against Children: Medico-Rituals and Assisted Reproductive Technologies in a Tuareg Couple's Quest for Parenthood." In Olsen and Sargent 2017, 69–89.

———. 2023. "Comparative Insights on Masking (or Not) in Coping with Covid-19: Customary Tuareg Covering Niger, Controversial Covering in the United States, and Their Broader Implications for Theories of Danger, Pollution, and Contagion." *Lidé mesta* 2: 139–70.

Renne, Elisha P. 2010. *The Politics of Polio in Northern Nigeria.* Bloomington: Indiana University Press.

———. 2017. "Ear Infections, Malnutrition, and Circuitous Health Care Treatments in Zaria, Nigeria." In Olsen and Sargent 2017, 187–206.

République du Niger. 1997. "Ordinance No. 97–002 du 10 janvier 1997 Portant Legislation Pharmaceutique."

Roberts, Jonathan. 2021. *Sharing the Burden of Sickness: A History of Healing and Medicine in Accra.* Bloomington: Indiana University Press.

Robertson, R. 2012. "Globalisation or glocalization?" *Journal of International Communication* 18 (2): 191–208.

Robinson, Cedric. 1983. *Black Marxism: The Making of the Black Radical Tradition.* London: Zed Press.

Rogers, Toby. 2024. "Involuntary Enclosure for All: Encapsulating the Human Body for the Purpose of Exploitation." *Review,* February 22–March 12, 2024, 3, 13–14.

Sams, Kelley. 2016. "A Medicine for every sickness: A visual reflection on the treatment of eye disease in rural Niger." *Medicine Anthropology Theory* 3 (2): 313–24.

———. 2017. "Engaging Conceptions of Identity in a Context of Medical Pluralism: Explaining Treatment Choices for Everyday Illness in Niger." *Sociology of Health & Illness* 39 (7): 1100–116.

———. 2022. Personal communication.

Sams, Kelley, and Tabitha Hrynick. 2020. *Tackling Deadly Diseases in Africa: Key Considerations for Epidemic Response and Preparedness in Niger.* DAI Global Health. Institute of Development Studies.

Sams, Kelley, Chiara Alfieri, Fleur Beauvieux, Frimin Kra, Carlotta Magnani, Francesca Mininel, and Sandrine Musso. 2021. "'. . . but not gagged': Responding to Covid-19 and its control measures in France, Italy, and the USA." *Anthropology Today* 37(6): 5–8.

Sargent, Carolyn, and James Leslie Kennell. 2017. "Elusive Paths, Fluid Care: Seeking Healing and Protection in the Republic of Benin." In Olsen and Sargent 2017, 227–43.

Schmoll, Pamela. 1993. "Black Stomach, Beautiful Stones: Soul-Eating Among Hausa in Niger." In *Modernity and Its Malcontents: Ritual and Power in Postcolonial Africa,* edited by Jean Comaraff and John Comaraff, 193–220. Chicago: University of Chicago Press.

Schoepf, Brooke Grundfest. 2017. "Medical Pluralism Revisited: A Memoir." In Olsen and Sargent 2017, 110–36.

Scoones, Ian. 2019. *What Is Uncertainty and Why Does It Matter?* STEPS Working Paper 105, Brighton, UK: STEPS Centre.

Scott, James C. 1985. *Weapons of the Weak: Everyday Forms of Peasant Resistance.* New Haven, CT: Yale University Press.

Sengul, Halil, and Arzu Bulut. 2020. "Determination of the relationship between physician trust, medical mistrust, and self-confidence in the health services provided in Turkey." *International Journal of Human Sciences* 17 (4): 1222–34.

Sidikou, Hamidou A. 1980. "Niamey, étude de géographie socio-urbaine." Thèse pour le Docto-rat, Université de Rouen Haute-Normandie.

Smith, Daniel Jordan. 2022. *Every Household Its Own Government: Improvised Infrastructure, Entrepreneurial Citizens, the State in Nigeria*. Princeton, NJ: Princeton University Press.

Smith, Mary F. 1954. *Baba of Karo: A Woman of the Muslim Hausa*. London: Faber and Faber.

Sounaye, Abdoulaye. 2013. "Alarama is all at once: preacher, media 'savvy', and religious entre-preneur in Niamey." *Journal of African Cultural Studies* 25 (1): 88–102.

Squibb, Eliza. 2022. Personal communication.

Stewart, Pamela, and Andrew Strathern. 2003. *Witchcraft, Sorcery, Rumors, Gossip*. Cambridge: Cambridge University Press.

Stoller, Paul. 1989. *Fusion of the Worlds: An Ethnography of Possession Among the Songhay of Niger*. Chicago: University of Chicago Press.

———. 2004. *Stranger in the Village of the Sick*. Boston: Beacon Press.

Stoller, Paul, and Cheryl Olkes. 1987. *In Sorcery's Shadow: A Memoir of Apprenticeship Among the Songhay of Niger*. Chicago: University of Chicago Press.

Stroeken, Koen. 2017. "The Individualization of Illness: Bewitchment and the Mental in Postco-lonial Tanzania." In Olsen and Sargent 2017, 151–69.

Sztompka, Piotr. 1999. *Trust: A Sociological Theory*. Cambridge: Cambridge University Press.

Taylor, Christopher C. 2017. "Ihahamuka—PTSD in Post-Genocidal Rwanda: Culture, Conti-nuity, and Change in Rwandan Therapeutics." In Olsen and Sargent 2017, 170–86. Bloom-ington: Indiana University Press.

Thurston, Alexander. 2018. *Boko Haram: The History of an African Jihadist Movement*. Prince-ton, NJ: Princeton University Press.

Tremearne, Arthur J. N. 1914. *The Ban of the Bori: Demons and Demon Dancing in West and North Africa*. London: Health, Cranton, and Ouseley.

Trovalla, Ulrika. 2017. "Wishful Doing: Journeying in a Nigerian Medical Landscape." In Olsen and Sargent 2017, 137–50.

Turner, Patricia A. 1993. *I Heard It Through the Grapevine: Rumor in African American Culture*. Berkeley: University of California Press.

Twumasi, Patrick A. 1979. "History of Pluralistic Medical Systems: A Sociological Analysis of the Ghanian Case." *Issue: A Journal of Opinion* 9 (3): 29–34.

UNICEF. 2019. "Niger." Accessed December 30, 2024. http://data.unicef.org > FGM_NER.

———. 2023. "UNICEF Data Warehouse." Accessed December 28, 2023. https://data.unicef.org/resources/data_explorer/unicef_f/?ag=UNICEF&df=GLOBAL_DATAFLOW&ver=1.0&dq=NER.IM_DTP3.&startPeriod=1970&endPeriod=2023.

United Nations (UN). 1948. The Universal Declaration of Human Rights.

United Nations Development Programme (UNDP). 2022. "Human Development Reports: Human Development Index (HDI)." Accessed February 23, 2023. https://hdr.undp.org/data-center/human-development-index#/indicies/HDI.)

van der Geest, Sjaak, and Susan Reynolds Whyte. 1999. "The Charm of Medicines: Metaphors and Metonyms." *Medical Anthropology Quarterly* New Series 3 (4): 345–67.

van der Geest, Sjaak, Susan Reynolds Whyte, and Anita Hardon. 1996. "The Anthropology of Pharmaceuticals: A Biographical Approach." *Annual Review of Anthropology* 25: 153–78.

Wall, L. Lewis. 1988. *Hausa Medicine: Illness and Well-Being in a West African Culture*. Durham, NC: Duke University Press.

White, Luise. 2000. *Speaking with Vampires: Rumor and History in Colonial Africa*. Berkeley: University of California Press.

Whyte, Susan Reynolds, Sjaak van der Geest, and Anita Hardon. 2002. *Social Lives of Medicines*. Cambridge: Cambridge University Press.

World Bank. 2022. "Fertility rate, total (births per woman)." Accessed November 13, 2023. https://data.worldbank.org/indicator/SP.DYN.TFRT.IN.

———. 2024. "Niger Overview." March 19, 2024. Accessed August 6, 2024. https://www.worldbank.org/en/country/niger/overview.

World Bank Group. 2023. "Niger Literacy." Accessed August 13, 2024. https://data.worldbank.org/indicator/SE.ADT.LITR.ZS?display=g&locations=NE.

World Health Organization. 2021. "Niger Report." Accessed December 25, 2023. https://www.who.int/about/accountability/results/who-results-report-2020-2021/country-profile/2021/niger-approved.

Worldwide Cancer Research. 2020. "Could somebody be hiding the cure for cancer?" March 25, 2020. Accessed August 5, 2024. https://www.worldwidecancerresearch.org/news-opinion/2020/march/could-somebody-be-hiding-the-cure-for-cancer/.

Yahaya, Nasir. 2023. "Strategizing Islamic Medicine Marketing Through Social Media: The Case of Northern Nigeria." In *Strategies and Applications of Islamic Entrepreneurship*, edited by Ahmad Rafiki, Alfatih Gessan Pananjung, and Muhammad Dharma Putra Nasution, 201–17. Hershey, PA: IGI Global.

Youngstedt, Scott M. 2013. *Surviving with Dignity: Hausa Communities of Niamey, Niger*. Lanham, MD: Lexington Books.

———. 2021. "*Akwaku*: The Itinerant Pharmaceutical Vendors of Niamey, Niger." *Material Culture* 53 (2): 1–22.

Figures and tables are indicated by page numbers followed by *fig.* and *tab.* respectively.

# ACKNOWLEDGMENTS

*Negotiating Mistrust* could not have come to fruition without the collaboration and participation of hundreds of Nigériens. Political scientist Rahmane Idrissa deserves credit for setting me on the path that eventually led to this book. I also benefited from several conversations with him about the project over the years in Niamey and online. Social anthropologists Alkassoum Alasmagui and Cheifou Idrissa were critically important collaborators throughout the ethnographic research at the heart of this book. They shared their knowledge of medical mistrust and medical pluralism with me through lengthy conversations as well as written reports. Alasmagui and Idrissa helped me to construct interview questions and conducted some of the interviews, and they collected more than 50 traditional and Islamic plant medicines. Koche "Yaji" Dan Jima was as an invaluable "gatekeeper" as he introduced me to healers, especially Islamic healers, that I never would have met on my own. He also helped me organize focus group discussions and consented to lengthy interviews on health, illness, and healing in Niger. Rabiou "Rabé" Dan Maradi informed me of the existence of Association des Tradi-Practiciens du Niger, accompanied me to their difficult-to-find office, and introduced me to the Board of Directors. He also shared personal details of his suffering and eclectic therapeutic trajectory involving all three medical sectors of Niger. Djibrilla Garba Kora and Lamine Garba Kora offered consistent friendly support, advice, and hospitality. Last but certainly not least, I sincerely thank the hundreds of Nigériens who consented to interviews and focus group participation for their patience, openness, and in many cases, willingness to share very personal health information.

I dedicate this book to Brian "Barké" Nowak, an ethnographer and humanitarian aid specialist who lived in Niger from 2005 until he was tragically killed there in 2021. Barké inspired me with his love and appreciation of Nigérien people and cultures and his enthusiastic willingness to share this and his deep knowledge with me. I learned much from Barké as he knew as much or more about traditional healing, music, and languages than any non-Nigérien, and even most Nigériens.

I gratefully acknowledge Saginaw Valley State University, my home institution, for trusting me with Faculty Research Grants to cover my travel to and from Niger and research and living costs in country for this project in 2017, 2018, 2019, 2021, 2022, and 2023 as well as granting me a sabbatical leave in the 2023–2024 academic year to complete the writing of this book.

I sincerely thank Elisabeth Maselli, senior editor at the University of Pennsylvania Press, for being a strong advocate for this project from beginning to end. Maselli offered valuable suggestions about the direction of the book, and her professionalism, efficiency, and enthusiasm reduced my stress significantly. I thank Alma Gottlieb, editor of the Contemporary Ethnography Series, for offering very detailed, constructive advice regarding theory, ethnography, and organization that strengthened the book. I also deeply appreciate the work of two anonymous reviewers for University of Pennsylvania Press. Their constructive suggestions, drawing from expertise in medical anthropology and deep knowledge of Niger, helped me focus my arguments and the organization of the book.

I am enormously grateful to Katherine Wiley, developmental editor at Goldenrod Editorial and Consulting. Other than the anonymous reviewers, only Wiley read drafts of each chapter. I am extremely fortunate to have worked with a highly skilled editor who is also an excellent writer and anthropologist of West Africa. She consistently offered timely and critical feedback on everything from clarifying individual sentences to "the big picture" arguments and structure. Perhaps most importantly, Wiley consistently encouraged me to write my book in the way that I wanted it written.

I thank Souleymane Diallo for inviting me to present my paper, "Traditional Healing in Niamey, Niger," at the University of Münster, Germany, in 2021. Diallo, Birgit Meyer, and others offered valuable insights. I am grateful to Ousmane Sène and Mariane Yade for inviting me to present an updated version of the paper, "Brassage and Change in Traditional Medicine in Niamey, Niger" at the West African Research Center in Dakar, Senegal, in 2022. I benefited greatly from the lively discussion that followed, and particularly the insightful commentary provided by Sène, Yade, Papa Mohamed Camara, and Boubé Namaiwa. Follow-up conversations with Namaiwa were stimulating and fruitful, particularly because he is a Nigérien professor working in

Dakar who has extensive knowledge of traditional medicine in Niger and of Nigérien traditional healers working in Dakar.

Many people read various drafts of parts of the book and offered valuable advice. Historian Jeff Kolnick helped me with the presentation of the history of medical pluralism and mistrust in Niger and immediately recognized the importance of the heat–cold complex. I knew that I wanted to include some discussion of heat–cold but he encouraged me to complete a chapter-length analysis of it. Medical anthropologists Conerly Casey and Kelley Sams graciously shared informed advice on many different drafts. Their input and encouragement were extremely useful. Casey and I co-organized a panel entitled "A Shifting Sahel: Ecologies of Health and Healing across Niger and Northern Nigeria" at the 2022 Annual Meeting of the American Anthropological Association in Seattle that included Susan J. Rasmussen, Paul Stoller, Adeline Masquelier, and Eliza Squibb. I learned much about health, illness, and healing in Niger and Northen Nigeria from their presentations and benefited from their comments on my paper that was focused on COVID-19 in Niger. I am especially appreciative of Squibb's advice. She creatively blends public health work with textile and visual arts in Niger and elsewhere and offered important suggestions over much of the trajectory of this project, including carefully reading multiple drafts and pointing me toward important sources. Pediatrician Laura Bledsoe, anthropologists Ali Heller, Laura Miller, and Tamara Turner, public health specialist Shelly Nicholson, and ethnomusicologist Eric Schmidt also offered useful advice.

I thank several colleagues at Saginaw Valley State University who offered important suggestions that strengthened this book. Robert S. Drew helped me navigate the proposal process and provided constructive advice on several segments of the book. Sara Beth Keough encouraged me to consider the material culture of medicine. Maureen Muchimba provided important ideas about medical pluralism in various parts of Africa. Jesse Donahue offered relevant reading suggestions. Anthropology students Charles Ferens and Christina Quigley provided useful feedback on my writing about street pharmaceutical vendors.

I sincerely thank development aid specialist Maggie Janes-Lucas for inviting me to stay in her home and use her car during research trips in 2018, 2019, 2021, and 2022. Her knowledge of health in Niger allowed her to offer helpful feedback, and her wonderful hospitality made me feel very welcome and comfortable. I am grateful to artist Issa Yacouba Oumarou for sharing his work on cultivating medicinal plants and finding a comfortable, centrally located villa to rent with political scientist William F. S. Miles in 2023. Miles provided stimulating comments on the project orally and in writing and shared his long-term nuanced knowledge of Nigérien cultures with me.

Jamila Youngstedt and Reid Youngstedt, my wonderful children, also inspired me. They have traveled to Niger multiple times with me and learned to appreciate Nigériens, patiently waited for me when I went alone, and have taught me to think about Nigériens from different perspectives.

I gratefully acknowledge the journal *Material Culture* for granting me permission to reprint portions of my article, "*Akwaku*: The Itinerant Pharmaceutical Vendors of Niamey, Niger," 53, no. 2 (2021): 1–22. These segments are located primarily in Chapter 5.